PRAISE FOR *ALL OF US WARRIORS*

"This book serves as a tremendous resource for cancer patients and their families. Their faith, strength, and perseverance should serve as an example for others facing adversity. They are an inspiration to many, including myself."
—**Ricardo J. Komotar, MD, FAANS, FACS,** Program Director, Department of Neurological Surgery, University of Miami School of Medicine

"This book is life-changing for cancer patients and their loved ones. It is like a conversation with a new best friend (or twenty of them), full of understanding, acceptance, and practical advice gained from personal experience. It opened a door that made me want to share my story and hear the stories of others. It demonstrates how much we each have to gain and to give within our unique community, and contains real information and strategies that cannot be found in online medical sites. It is, simply, a powerful fuel for the body and the soul."
—**Doris Schneider,** breast cancer survivor and author of *Borrowed Things, By Way of Water,* and *Nana and the "c"*

"The word 'cancer' can be a frightening term to many. *All Of Us Warriors: Cancer Stories of Survival And Loss* strips away the fear, demonstrating time and again that there is always hope and there can be joy in life, even when one is faced with the tremendous challenges of illness."
—**Dr. Robin Williams,** breast surgeon at Saint Thomas Medical Partners

"What a great book of stories—true stories of persistence, patience, and determination. I highly recommend it for any family with a cancer diagnosis."

—**Dr. Peter R. Ledoux**, breast surgeon at PRMA

"To see that you are not alone is a great comfort. Rebecca Munn has presented twenty stories for you to read with elements of shock, disbelief, and debility of the fight, but each case brings some new elements to consider. Cancer is a hard thing to accept; reading these stories will help."

—**R. Scott Anderson, MD, FACR**, medical director of Anderson Regional Cancer Center and author of *The Hard Times* and *Terrence and the Toilet Fairy*

Love always

In my Prayers each Day

All of Us
WARRIORS

Ma -

All of Us
WARRIORS

CANCER
STORIES *of*
SURVIVAL
and LOSS

Rebecca Whitehead Munn

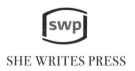

SHE WRITES PRESS

Published 2020
Printed in the United States of America
Print ISBN: 978-1-63152-795-1
E-ISBN: 978-1-63152-796-8
Library of Congress Control Number: 2020905837

For information, address:
She Writes Press
1569 Solano Ave #546
Berkeley, CA 94707

Interior design by Tabitha Lahr

She Writes Press is a division of SparkPoint Studio, LLC.

DEDICATION

————•—●—•————

This book is dedicated to my mother, who survived late-stage breast cancer in her fifties and later lost the battle to colon cancer in her seventies. She was an invaluable role model for me in living and in dying.

This book is also dedicated to the people who were willing to speak up and bare all on these pages, in an effort to demystify the cancer experience and help others: Melissa, Robyn, Helen, Ronn, Jennifer, Bill K., Dana, Bill G., Valerie, Dan, Peggy, Robert, Holly, Nikki, Kim, Gina, Tricia, Debi, Alan, and Kristi.

CONTENTS

FOREWORD

————•—●—•————

C ancer impacts each of us. One-point-seven million men and women will be diagnosed with cancer this year, and nearly two out of every five people will be diagnosed with cancer in their lifetime. Individuals, families, friends, and colleagues are all impacted by cancer. What used to be never discussed is now a familiar topic.

Fortunately, major advances in treatment are leading to patients living longer and better. Cancers that were untreatable twenty years ago are now routinely treated. The goal of finding a cure has not changed, but where we cannot achieve cure, we are striving to reduce cancer and the symptoms that come from it—allowing individuals to live with cancer. And as treatments become more effective, they are increasingly less harmful, allowing individuals to live with quality.

Innovations in technology and deeper scientific insights have led to the discovery of novel treatments that can specifically target cancer cells, and not healthy cells. As well, breakthroughs in our understanding of how the immune system can be used to identify and kill cancer have led to the development of groundbreaking approaches in cancer treatment that have revolutionized the landscape of cancer care. We are experiencing one of the greatest eras of achievement in cancer treatment, and the future is brighter than ever.

But it hasn't always been this way. Growing up with a father who worked as an oncologist allowed me to see the challenges of caring for patients with cancer. The availability of therapies was more limited; and these treatments were often toxic, with modest benefits. My father's partners discouraged me from going into oncology. Work would be hard, medicine would be increasingly regulated, and there were other pursuits that offered easier paths in life. My dad never pushed medicine on me, but he always supported my interest. I accompanied him on hospital rounds, spent summers in the lab and in the hospital, and shadowed different kinds of doctors to see all of the ways one could practice medicine. The one thing that always resonated with me was the gratitude patients and families had, even when things didn't turn out well. That gratitude convinced me that caring for others, even when they are at the hardest times in their lives, was a privileged role.

Oncology is a field where your impact is meaningful. Helping someone and their family through one of the hardest periods in their life is an honor. And to be able to provide hope, because advances in care are occurring at a rapid pace, is truly rewarding. Those advances come from research and the sacrifices of other patients and families. We still have far to go to help more people, and yet the successes of the past several years provide a foreshadowing that we will make even greater progress in the years ahead.

There is reason to have hope. I believe you will find inspiration and hope in each of the stories included in this book. The one truth of all cancer experiences is it will change your life, forever. The change may be small or unnoticeable or it may be life-threatening. These stories provide examples of why there is always hope for anyone fighting cancer and why that journey will not be taken alone.

—David R. Spigel, MD
　　Chief Scientific Officer
　　Director, Lung Cancer Research Program
　　Sarah Cannon Research Institute, a division of HCA Healthcare

INTRODUCTION

———•—●—•———

As I sat on my bed, propped up with pillows against the wall, the phone rang. It was a Thursday night in the spring of 1984, and I was reviewing my notes for my marketing test. I answered the phone and heard my mom's voice. It was a welcome distraction from my studying, although I could hear the uneasiness as she said hello. I put my book down and sat up, shifting my full attention to her voice. I can still remember that moment as if it were yesterday. I thought she would say hello quickly, as she had done many times before, and check in on my schoolwork, but as she started to speak, her words filled me with fear. Mom said, "Rebecca, I'm calling to let you know that I saw the doctor today. I was having some pain trying to raise my right arm. The appointment happened so fast, and he ran a bunch of tests. I was there all day and am exhausted. I need to tell you that I have been diagnosed with late-stage breast cancer." I was speechless as she continued to tell me more, struggling to process all the details she had just shared. The tests showed a tumor the size of a grapefruit on top of her right breast. The cancer was fairly advanced, as it had spread to most of the lymph nodes on her right side. Even with the advanced stage of cancer in her body, she said she was not really experiencing any symptoms. That was my mom—always focusing on everyone else's needs first and not paying attention to her own body. "My doctor wants to act quickly and has scheduled surgery for tomorrow at Methodist Hospital," she went on. "I would like you and your sisters to come to Houston, although I know that will be hard to manage. I'm going to be okay. I love you."

Although I struggled to get words out to respond to the news I had just heard, I managed to tell her how much I loved her and hung up. I tossed and turned in my bed through the night, thinking of my mom while my heart raced and chills rolled up and down my spine. As each hour passed, my body became more exhausted while my mind actively considered what this really meant for me. I realized around two a.m. that I had taken my mother for granted. I had learned to count on her always being there, and this news caught me totally by surprise. I wondered, *What will happen next? Is Mom really capable of surviving this illness, which sounds very serious?* My body froze as fear permeated every cell. My palms became sweaty, and my stomach turned over and over, like waves crashing on a beach. After a while, I instinctively put one hand on my stomach and one hand on my heart, calming my soul and enabling me to fall back asleep. The next day, I awoke in what felt like a haze, wondering if it had all been a dream. When I talked to my sister, I knew it was real. We both looked at each other in disbelief. This was my new reality—my mom had been diagnosed with cancer.

My sister and I discussed our schedules and determined that we could leave Austin a little after lunch for the two-and-a-half hour drive home to Houston. I called my teachers to let them know my situation and that I would be missing classes. After our morning classes, my sister and I drove to Houston to be with Mom and planned to stay through the following week. On that Friday at five o'clock, we arrived at our childhood home, just a few blocks from the Texas Medical Center and Methodist Hospital, where Mom had had her surgery earlier that day. Shortly thereafter, we went to the hospital to get an update. The doctor reported the procedure had gone well. He had been able to remove the tumor on her right breast. Because of the advanced stage of her cancer, he had also removed seventeen lymph nodes in her right armpit. I went into Mom's room and wrapped my arms around her, in between the oxygen and IV tubing. She was groggy from the anesthesia, although she smiled when she saw me.

"Mom, it's such a relief to see you! I imagine you are worn out." I took a breath as the reality of seeing her in her post-surgery state settled into my mind. I continued, "Mom, I will come back tomorrow to spend more time. I know you will be okay. I love you so much!" Her eyes lit up and then closed again as she dozed off.

Over the next few days, my sisters and I took turns going to visit Mom at Methodist Hospital, where she was recovering from surgery. Each of us was still a little numb from the news and somewhat withdrawn from the reality facing us. While we were all focused on Mom, we also realized how dependent our dad had become on her. On Saturday, while I was at the hospital and one of my sisters was home taking a nap, my dad went to wake her up. She was startled and worried that something else had happened to Mom, until she learned that he expected her to make his lunch, just as Mom had done day in and day out on the weekends before.

As I walked into Mom's room on that Saturday, I found her lying in her hospital bed, looking peaceful and yet exhausted. She grinned from ear to ear when she saw me, and energy seemed to flood her body. My heart filled with joy to see that she was indeed ok, as I had been concerned since seeing her briefly the night before. I ran over and hugged her, carefully avoiding the various tubes, as tears rolled down my cheeks. For what seemed like hours, I held on tight, like a little girl afraid of the dark. Finally, I kissed her on the cheek, sat next to her on her bed, and asked her to share what the experience had felt like to her. Despite the reality that she had learned only two days earlier of the cancerous tumor and had come through a difficult surgery, Mom wanted to move forward and focus quickly on her healing, versus talking about her surgery. She surprised me with her first request. She asked that I help her healing process. She wanted to teach me something about visualizing her body being healed. Although that concept was quite confusing to me at the time, it was typical of my mom to want to move forward and focus on the positive, despite her circumstances. I also knew how strongly she believed in the power of her mind and its capacity for healing her body. I took a deep breath as a little voice inside me told me to be open to her request and follow her wishes. Here was a chance for me to give back to her, as she had done countless times for me before. She said, "Rebecca, I know it is possible for me to survive this cancer. I am much stronger than any disease. Every minute I have been lying here in this hospital bed following my surgery, I have been focusing my attention on healing. And now I want a little of your help."

Mom's conviction that her mind could heal her body stemmed in part from her study of the book *Love, Medicine, and Miracles*, by Bernie Siegel, and in part from her grandmother Dora Annetta, who had been a healer during Mom's childhood, catching rainwater and making homeopathic treatments for ailments. Mom approached her healing from her cancer surgery much as Dora Annetta would have, with persistence and determination. As I sat there in her hospital room, now a willing participant, Mom instructed me: "Now, focus all of your mind and attention on the affected area up here on my right breast, and imagine the cancer cells evaporating like water on a hot, sunny day." I closed my eyes and tried to visualize exactly what she asked. We sat there for what felt like hours with our eyes closed, trying to keep our attention focused on picturing the cancer dissolving.

As I practiced this new skill, my mind wandered a bit. I thought about things that dissolve or fade away in nature. I loved welcoming the spring flowers after the frozen hibernation of the ground in winter. One of my favorite things to do as a little girl was to pick a stem of goatsbeard wildflowers with the seed head still intact. I would hold a bloom in my hand, close my eyes, and make a wish, and then open my eyes and blow the white seeds away.

Each stem would disappear one at a time, carried off by the wind. As I thought of this experience, I decided that would be another way for me to visualize Mom's body healing. I sat there in silence with my eyes closed, holding her hand, and visualizing the cancer cells being those seed stems. I made a wish for healing and then blew the seeds away, imagining the wind taking them to a faraway place outside Mom's body. It calmed my heart to be doing my part in assisting Mom's healing, and she was calmed by my willingness to participate, learn, and help her survive. Day after day, even after she was released from the hospital, Mom sustained her focus on healing her body on her own and with my help.

After I went back to Austin to resume my college classes, I thought of her each night before I went to bed, and I continued to practice these visualizations. As Mom endured chemotherapy and radiation weekly for the next six months, she suffered many of the humiliating and uncomfortable side effects, including hair loss, swollen ankles, and an upset stomach. While wigs are very common today, and organizations like Locks of Love enable healthy people to donate hair for wigs, they were very hard to find in 1984. We were fortunate to live in Houston, where Mom had access to wigs through MD Anderson Cancer Center. She also reached out to her friends to support her and help her process the physical and emotional impacts of the cancer. She started taking daily walks with these friends around her neighborhood and around Rice University's campus, near our childhood home. Her friends provided a safe place and supportive ear for Mom to release her anger and sadness about the cancer and the changes she was experiencing in her body.

Her face always lit up when she talked about those walks and how much her friends buoyed her. In doing so, Mom modeled for me how valuable ongoing encouragement and love from close friends is to lifelong health. Around the time I graduated from college, Mom successfully completed her chemotherapy and radiation treatments and moved into remission with grace and reverence.

Her hair grew back gray and wavy—a big change from the coal-black, straight hair we had known growing up. Since the cancer was late stage and had spread to so many of her lymph nodes, the medical protocol was to check her body regularly to make sure the cancer did not show up again. So, for fifteen years following the official start of her remission, Mom endured painful bone marrow and liver tests every six months. She would go off quietly to those appointments, without ever drawing attention to the experience, the pain she endured, or the process. She was so very strong and determined to live a long life and share it with the people she loved, minimizing any discomfort or pain she may have been feeling.

At the time of her surgery, Mom's doctor had shared with her the appropriate amount of information about her tumor: where it was and what kind of operation he would perform, including removing many of the lymph nodes under her right arm. However, he had stopped short of telling her the odds of her surviving. At the time, I had been so overwhelmed with the shock of what was happening that I had not thought to ask. When I reflected on it later, my interpretation was that he must have believed her situation was tenuous enough, amid all the surgery and treatments, that giving her odds of surviving would not have added anything positive to her outlook or her healing process. At the time, we all fully trusted this physician and his choices and believed he knew best about what he did and didn't share. What he did explain to each of us was how advanced a level her cancer had reached, and that it had a 98 percent chance of recurrence. He also mentioned that because Mom's own mother had died of breast cancer, each of us, her five daughters, had a 75 percent chance of being diagnosed with breast cancer ourselves.

Mom lived a cancer-free full live for seventeen years until she was diagnosed with colorectal cancer in 2003. Following her diagnosis, she started treatment with traditional Western methods—radiation and chemotherapy, followed by surgery—but she quickly felt in her body that while that regimen was killing the cancer cells, the drugs were also killing her healthy cells. She suffered many of the debilitating side effects of this chemotherapy drug, including mouth sores, diarrhea, and dry eyes. After her surgery, she was only able to withstand a portion of her post-surgery chemotherapy treatments. A year and a half later, when she discovered the cancer had metastasized into her lungs, she was determined to have a good quality of life for whatever time she had left. She tried a chemotherapy regimen, although it made her deeply ill again, and she almost died from low potassium. Mom stopped her chemotherapy infusions and switched to taking Chinese herbs daily and having weekly acupuncture treatments. She lived fairly comfortably for another year and a half using these Eastern medicine techniques, in addition to taking daily walks around her neighborhood on Lake Austin.

Mom taught me so very much, both in her fruitful living years and in her last year on Earth. She was a voracious reader, always questioning the status quo and expanding her traditional faith to incorporate more metaphysical beliefs. My parents enjoyed a loving marriage for fifty-five years. Their marriage ended when my mother passed away in 2006 at age seventy-seven, when I was forty-three. Even in dying, she gave me an eye-opening and heartfelt opportunity to learn from her views. One important lesson she taught me through the process was that we don't really have to say good-bye to our loved ones as they pass from physical life. Rather, as they transition and take on the form of angels, they remain engaged in our lives by watching over us, cheering us on through our many joys, and supporting us through our tribulations. And sometimes, if we are open to believing it is possible, our loved ones boldly make themselves known and forever change our physical lives for the better.

• • •

In November of 2017, five months after I published my award-winning debut memoir about walking the end-of-life path with my mom, *The Gift of Goodbye: A Story of Agape Love*, I was working on my second manuscript. It was an expansion of one of my first book's themes, living an authentic life. I was practicing meditation and sitting in the peaceful space of my home one morning. I had just learned about a friend's cancer diagnosis—stage IV colon cancer for a woman in her early forties with three children under the age of eleven. I was heartbroken by this news and praying for grace and guidance. As I sat quietly, I heard a voice say, *You ought to write about these stories from the front lines of those living with and surviving cancer.* I looked around a little startled, confirming I was by myself, as my daughter had already left for school. As I sat with this idea, memories of all of I had learned of what had been helpful in my experiences with Mom came flooding back. The nuances of how to approach someone you love living with cancer, and the tips and tricks of helping others feel joy amid pain. I picked up my notebook and started jotting down questions I might ask if I was going to interview cancer survivors. Excitement pulsed through my veins as I considered how helpful it might be to others—to write the stories of those who have experienced a cancer diagnosis. And in that moment, I decided to shift my focus to try to demystify cancer through capturing stories from United States-based survivors and loved ones, men and women with different types of cancers and stages of the disease. Hearing of a loved one's or friend's diagnosis invokes such fear that it is hard to think clearly or know what to do next. And yet, at the time of writing this book, the incidence of cancer continues to rise globally, and current United States statistics include the following:

- In 2018, an estimated 1,735,350 new cases of cancer will be diagnosed in the United States and 609,640 people will die from the disease.
- The most common cancers (listed in descending order, according to estimated new cases in 2018) are breast cancer, lung and bronchial cancer, prostate cancer, colon and rectal cancer, melanoma of the skin, bladder cancer, non-Hodgkin's

lymphoma, kidney and renal pelvis cancer, endometrial cancer, leukemia, pancreatic cancer, thyroid cancer, and liver cancer.

- The number of new cases of cancer (cancer incidence) is 439.2 per 100,000 men and women per year (based on 2011–2015 cases).
- The number of cancer deaths (cancer mortality) is 163.5 per 100,000 men and women per year (based on 2011–2015 deaths).
- Cancer mortality is higher among men than women (196.8 per 100,000 men and 139.6 per 100,000 women). When comparing groups based on race/ethnicity and sex, cancer mortality is highest in African American men (239.9 per 100,000) and lowest in Asian/Pacific Islander women (88.3 per 100,000).
- In 2016, there were an estimated 15.5 million cancer survivors, a number that is expected to increase to 20.3 million by 2026.
- Based on data from 2013–2015, approximately 38.4 percent of men and women will be diagnosed with cancer at some point during their lifetimes.

Source: National Cancer Institute, www.cancer.gov

I had all these ideas swirling in my head when I happened to have lunch with Robyn, a dear friend who is a cancer survivor. Suddenly, it all fell into place. Together, we could write this story, of the journey of various cancer survivors and their advice. Between us, we connected with our friendship circle to find volunteers willing to participate in this book and share their stories. I have included the first half of Robyn's story below, how she discovered she had cancer. The rest of her story is in the first chapter.

Robyn's Story

It was a freezing night in Castle Rock, Colorado, and I was sleeping soundly next to my husband on January 28, 2016. All of a sudden, I woke up and began to rub my neck. As my hand moved down to the top of my left breast, I felt it. A lump the size of a grape was protruding out of my chest. Shocked by my new discovery, I immediately jumped out of bed, went into the kitchen, and started feeling all over my breasts for other lumps. Standing there alone in the kitchen, my stomach was turning upside down, and I could feel my heart pounding in my chest. *What is happening?* I wondered. Feeling unsettled and not sure what exactly was going on, I stared down at my chest again, hoping it would be gone and was just a dream. As I rubbed my fingers over the small protrusion on my breast that had not been there the day before, I decided, *Okay, this is probably a cyst. Cancer doesn't run in my family.* I took a deep breath and remembered it was two a.m.

I stumbled back to our room and fell into bed, convinced it was nothing to worry about. As I glanced next to me at my sleeping husband, memories flooded my mind of the trials we had weathered together several years earlier, testing the foundation of our relationship to its limits. For the first time in a couple of years, our life with three young children was on cruise control. I was working for my pastor in Denver and loved having the balance of working part time and being home with the kids. I decided not to wake my husband, as he was traveling to Salt Lake City for work in a few hours and needed rest. I was able to fall back asleep after breathing deeply for a while.

I woke up early the next morning, anxious about my son being sick and knowing I needed to get him to the doctor. I looked at my husband and said, as we both got out of bed, "Hey, babe, I found something last night, I need you to look at it." I pulled my sleep shirt aside so he could see.

"Oh, babe, I wouldn't worry about it. You're going to the doctor soon, so just wait and see what they say." We both agreed it was nothing serious. Never in our wildest dreams did we think in that moment of what might unfold in the coming months and years.

"Have a great trip, baby, I love you so much," I said as we hugged and kissed good-bye. The mom role in me kicked into high gear, despite my sleep deprivation. I moved to the closet to pull on my yoga pants and sweatshirt and slip into my UGGs.

I walked down the hall and stepped quietly into my son's room to wake him up. "Good morning baby, how are you feeling? Your head feels a little warm." He opened one eye and whispered that he didn't feel better, and then closed it again. I had made a doctor's appointment for him the day before in case he was still feeling ill today. I helped him out of bed and drove over to his doctor appointment with him. We arrived at the doctor's office and took a seat in the "sick" waiting area. The nurse called us back to the exam room, and I helped my son onto the table. The nurse took his temperature and checked his blood pressure as we talked about his symptoms. While he was down the hall getting an X-ray, I found his doctor and asked if she would mind looking at my new discovery.

She rubbed her fingers over the lump in several directions then looked up at me and said, "So I am thinking it would be good to go get this checked out right away, you know, just to make sure." I could read the look of concern on her face, which made me think it might be something. Just then, my son and the nurse walked back in with the X-ray. The X-ray showed signs of pneumonia in his lungs, which meant he would not be going back to school soon. We thanked her and left with a prescription. When we got home, I gave him some orange juice and helped him upstairs to his bed. As I left his room, my focus was now able to shift to me and what I would do next.

I picked up my phone and dialed my doctor's number, asking for the nurse. I got her voice mail and left a message, describing what I had found. She called back in about thirty minutes to ask how I was doing and said I would need a mammogram soon, probably before the one that was scheduled in two weeks. As we talked more about the details, she likely heard the concern in my voice and said she would have the doctor fax over an order right away. I thanked her and hung up. About fifteen minutes later, my phone rang. It was the imaging center calling to schedule the diagnostic mammogram. I was able to get an appointment the following Tuesday. Having the appointment set was a step toward answers, toward learning more, and I felt a little peace in my heart.

I made some tea and sat on the couch for a minute as the memory of what I had discovered in the night came flooding back. I closed my eyes and sat with this feeling, asking God to reveal what I needed to know. I opened my eyes and looked around the room taking in my space in the silence, imagining what might happen next. One thing I knew for sure was my life, our life as a family, would be forever changed if this were something serious. I closed my eyes and rubbed my fingers over the mass again. Yes, it was still there. I knew instinctively that God had woken me up that morning to show me what I needed to see. From this moment forward, I felt like His hand was on me, guiding the process.

I went upstairs to check on my son. I sat on his bed and put my arm around him as he sipped the orange juice. His eyes closed, and I set down the orange juice as I inched my way a little more on his bed, lying down next to him with my arm around him. My lack of sleep caught up with me, and I dozed off for a while. The sound of my girls talking and moving around the house downstairs woke me up. I gingerly slid out of my son's bed, making sure he stayed asleep, and went downstairs. All of a sudden, I heard the garage door opening and knew it was my husband home from his trip. I jumped up and greeted him at the back door, delighted to feel his arms wrapped around me. We hugged for a minute, and I updated him on our son's pneumonia, careful not to mention what the doctor had said about my discovery, as the girls were nearby.

Later that evening, when the kids were in their rooms and we could talk privately, I shared the update from the doctor about my lump and my upcoming mammogram appointment. We both felt some relief knowing that the next step in a plan was set.

On Monday, I called my friend and asked her to meet me in the parking lot after school. I shared the details of my discovery, and that I was scared and wanted her opinion. She came to my mind as she had survived breast cancer ten years before. My younger daughter and her daughter were best friends. I felt at ease around her and knew she would be able to give me good advice, as she had experienced a cancer diagnosis and treatment. That afternoon, we each drove to school, picked up our kids, and pulled into parking spaces next to each other. "Hey kids, y'all get out and say hi," I said to my kids. They jumped out of the car as she walked over to me.

She got in the car, leaned over, and felt the lump. "Honestly, I don't like the way this feels, but we need to confirm it with tests. I am glad you are going in tomorrow for a mammogram. I'm here for you, Robyn, call anytime with any question." We hugged, and I thanked her for being there for me, offering to support me. Knowing she was right that this mass was concerning, I felt both validated and comforted by her support. As I walked through the next steps of the discovery process, she was a source of comfort and my trusted authority as I learned each new piece of information.

The next day came quickly with the busyness of taking care of my three kids, the day of my mammogram appointment. My mother-in-law had insisted on going with me. My husband had a big meeting, and I didn't want him to miss it. As I went back into the scanning room, I was feeling peaceful, as my mother-in-law waited outside. I showed the technician where the lump was. She took several images of both breasts and a few extra of my left one. She recommended I wait for the radiologist to read the scan. I went back to the waiting room and sat next to my mother-in-law on the couch. I tried to distract myself and flipped through pages in a magazine as two hours went by. The anxiety kicked in, as the wait had never taken that long before. Finally, my name was called.

We went back as the nurse ushered us into a different room with a bed and a machine next to it. I could feel instinctively that this was not good. She said, "The radiologist did see the mass on the film and wants you to have an ultrasound." I hyper-focused on what was going to happen next and felt a little out of my body, as if I was an observer in my story. As I walked over to lie down on the table, I still didn't believe it was cancer. As the technician rolled the probe over my left breast, I could see the mass on the screen. It looked like a tree branch. Tears started rolling down my cheeks, and I felt frightened, imagining that it was probably cancer. I looked at the technician and asked, "What do you see?"

She looked at me and said, "I am going to get the radiologist. I want him to see it."

I called my sister four times and kept leaving messages, "Where are you? I need you!" The technician returned with the radiologist and showed him the images. He looked at me and said, "I would recommend you make an appointment for a biopsy." All of a sudden, the words settled into my mind, and I began to cry hysterically. I looked at him and said I was not getting off the table until he performed the biopsy, right there. I wanted answers as quickly as I could get them and was determined not to wait. I didn't care if I was inconveniencing anyone. I wanted to know what was going on and wanted to know now.

The radiologist said he would see what he could do and left. He returned a few minutes later with a nurse and said he was able to move some other appointments. I found out later that the nurse had been about to go out on lunch break and could see how upset I was. The nurse had told the radiologist that she would stay to help, which enabled him to perform the biopsy at that time. The nurse stood by my side and held my hand as the radiologist prepared my breast for the biopsy. She had a warm presence about her and a calming smile. I felt relaxed in her presence and my heart filled with peace, and then my eyes caught her badge. Just above her picture was a sticker that said, "I love Jesus." All of a sudden, the muscles in my tense shoulders began to relax, and my heart rate slowed down from its racing pace. It felt like she was an angel sent from God. She exuded unconditional love and was so compassionate. She made sure I was taken care of and was selfless and gentle in her demeanor.

Two days later, on February 5th, I was at the school in the afternoon to watch my daughters play in their volleyball game. I could feel my phone vibrating in my pocket, and as I pulled it out, I quickly recognized the number. It was the doctor. I stepped out of the gym as I pressed the green button on my phone to answer. The radiologist confirmed that the mass was cancerous. He also recommended I have more scans and more biopsies to check my lymph nodes. I stood there as I hung up, feeling chills run up my spine and wondering if this was real. *Did I really just hear the words, you have cancer?* I wandered a little aimlessly back into the gym, found my mother-in-law, and said, "Will you come outside for a minute with me? I need to talk to you." She followed me out into the hallway, noticing the concern that covered my face. I grabbed her hands and said, "I need you to stay here. I just got confirmation that I have cancer and need to go outside." A look of shock brushed over her face as she wrapped her arms around me. I was in shock, feeling scared, and still not believing the words I had just heard. *You have cancer.* I was pacing the floor, looking out the window for my husband. He called a couple of minutes later as he was pulling up. I told him to stay in the car and I would be right there.

I got in the car, looked over at him and said, "The doctor just called and confirmed that I have stage II-B breast cancer." A waterfall of tears started pouring down our cheeks as we sat there, arms wrapped around each other, both processing this news and what it meant for us and our three kids. After a few minutes, I looked outside and remembered that we were in the school parking lot, and there was a volleyball game happening inside. Thinking of my family shifted my focus to attack mode, and I knew it was time for a game plan. I said, "I'm calling my doctor tomorrow, and we are going to take care of this. I need you to stay here with the kids, and I am going home." He leaned over and kissed me as we sobbed some more, the news still penetrating through our hearts.

As I drove home, I called both my sister and my best friend and shared the news with each of them. I felt supported by their kind words and grateful for the willingness of each of them to walk this journey with me, step by step. I was thankful that my sister lived in Denver, near me, as I knew her support would be crucial in having another ear at the many doctors' appointments that were to come. As I heard my husband's car pull into the garage, I needed to pull myself together. I had learned from previous situations how to hide my emotions. One of my main goals was to protect the kids from any sadness I had faced. We had decided that we would tell the kids that evening. It felt like a terrible dream, knowing that they would have to walk through a scary time at their young age.

He put his arm around me, and then told our children that I had been diagnosed with breast cancer. He did his best to stay positive, saying that we had good doctors and would get through it together. Watching each of their faces as they heard that I had cancer was one of the worst experiences of my life. They were in total disbelief. I could see concern and fear painted over their faces. None of us really knew what it meant to hear those words, that Mom has cancer. My heart was breaking in two as I watched tears stream down their faces. I knew I had to hold it together for them, reassure them that I would get through this. I believed it, and I knew it. My goal was to help them feel comfortable in talking about their feelings. I sat back as I watched each of them process this news; wanting to take away the fear I could see in their eyes. The feeling of protection that came over me was all encompassing. I most wanted to change our circumstances and make the reality of my cancer diagnosis go away for them. My sadness deepened as I knew I couldn't. Then my thoughts turned to my husband and what he was going to experience as we walked this path, and I endured treatment. I've never been good at receiving, and here we were, facing a strenuous and unknown path, one that would require me to let go and receive.

The next morning, I felt a strong surge to take action, build a plan, and know what was going to happen next. I talked to my doctor about the tests I needed, and I was able to get an appointment with a surgeon at a local hospital for the following Monday, February 9th. The earliest I was able to get in for the additional tests at the hospital was Wednesday, February 11th. I worked through all of the test scheduling and hung up. Despite the heaviness I felt in my heart regarding my diagnosis, I was able to return to a somewhat normal routine, given that we had appointments lined up, and a plan was forming. Life raising three young children consumed my focus for the days leading up to the appointments and testing.

On Monday, I met with the surgeon at a local hospital, and she shared the news that I had triple negative breast cancer, which is not a hormone-fed type of cancer. I sat there as I felt my stomach drop, knowing this was a tough type of cancer to recover from. As the reality of what these words meant started to settle in, my heart started racing. Tears poured down my cheeks as my husband wrapped his arm around me. I couldn't believe it. The one thing I do remember is that it was very important for me to have the BRACA 1 and BRACA 2 blood test, which determines if this type of cancer is hereditary. It was most important for me to know if my girls were at risk. Fortunately, the test came back negative for both of the BRACA genes.

I instinctively felt I needed a second opinion. I picked up my phone and called a leading cancer center near where my dad lives to set up appointments and felt grateful that they would be able to see me the week of February 16th. As the nurses and technicians poked and prodded me all day on the 11th, I knew I was one step closer to having all the information I needed to finalize my plan. When I left the hospital, exhausted from a long day, the nurse said I would hear the results in a day or two.

On Friday, February 13th, I was sitting with my husband having lunch when the doctor called. It was my forty-sixth birthday. I answered the phone and heard my doctor share what he had learned from the tests. Sadly, the news was that my lymph nodes also contained cancer cells. I hung up and told my husband. We held hands as tears rolled down my cheeks. He said, "Babe, we are going to get through this, one step at a time. I am here, whatever you need. We will walk this road, side by side." We stared at each other for a while as my mind raced forward to what would happen next. Likely I would endure more tests and scans and learn about treatment plans and timing.

• • •

With the increasing incidence of cancer in our world and close to 40 percent of people getting a cancer diagnosis in their lifetime, each of us will be touched in some way by this disease, either through a personal diagnosis or through learning of a loved one, friend, or colleague in the community with a diagnosis. Each cancer story is unique in many ways, as you saw in my story and Robyn's above. My goal in how I architected the stories in this book was to present a realistic face of cancer—the highs and lows, the good and bad, the surviving and sometimes the inevitable reality of dying. And while these stories include the transparent, sometimes grueling, details of the treatment process, each story is inspirational in some way and includes growth through loss, whether a loss of a body part or more. The stories also engender hope and have a thread of positivity woven throughout.

Robyn and I interviewed sixteen men and women from five different states in the US, who were diagnosed with seven different types of cancer ranging from breast to brain to lymphoma to colon to lung, and in stages I to IV. I have included how each person found out and how each person told their loved ones, what each of them experienced as they walked their treatment path, what was helpful and what was not, and what advice they have for others. While I captured themes in each story, I also learned a valuable lesson: That a cancer diagnosis and the resulting treatment and experience are an "n" of one, meaning each story is unique to that individual, even if it is the same type and stage of cancer. In an effort to bring a balanced perspective of cancer, I have also included a story from a man whose wife fought four years and lost the battle to melanoma and a woman whose husband was diagnosed with small cell carcinoma and died within a year. I have included a perspective from two oncologists as well, one in the Foreword and one in the Epilogue, as physicians are an integral component of a cancer story.

My hope is that these twenty stories, including the one below, serve as an inspirational guide for an individual with a cancer diagnosis or going through treatment, or for anyone whose friend, coworker, or loved one has just been diagnosed. The common message through all of the stories is to love through the fear and to engage, versus withdraw or give others "space". An important note about each story: I have purposefully removed the last names, the names of family members, friends, doctors, imaging centers, and health systems in order to keep the focus on the individual's story.

The idea for writing this book was born out of praying for my friend Melissa, also known as Isse, following her colon cancer diagnosis. I am honoring her by sharing her letter to the editor of the Nashville paper, *The Tennessean*. My hope is her story will help you take any potential symptoms seriously and have them checked out.

"I discovered colon cancer too late, but I want to make sure you don't"

by Melissa Waddey
April 3, 2019

My symptoms were easy to explain away. Exhaustion? I had just gotten a promotion. Weight loss? I was running myself ragged. Nausea? Too much grease in my diet. And the blood in my stool for the past several years? Internal hemorrhoids, my doctors assured me, very common in women who've had children.

But the consequences of ignoring your body when it's trying to tell you something can be hard. In my case, they were the hardest imaginable. In November 2017—after I finally scheduled the colonoscopy I was told I didn't need due to my young age—I learned I had stage IV colon cancer.

I will live with this horrific disease the rest of my days. Those days will be fewer than my loving husband, three beautiful young children, and I want them to be. I had to resign my new position as the first woman group president, ambulatory and operations services, of LifePoint Health. And I spend far too much of my precious time at hospitals or resting at home, my energy completely depleted at only forty-three years old.

Yet today, I have a stronger sense of God's purpose for me than I've had before. I am determined to save lives, to use every ounce of my strength to urge people to recognize the warning signs of colon cancer and take action—no matter how young you are or how squeamish you might be about bodily functions.

That's why I teamed up with my wonderful former colleagues from LifePoint Health to bring Get Your Rear in Gear, a family-friendly 5K walk/run, to Nashville for the first time on March 9, 2019. I am delighted to report we exceeded all expectations for an inaugural fundraiser, drawing more than a thousand participants and raising over $150,000.

Get Your Rear in Gear events are orchestrated across the country during March, which is Colon Cancer Awareness Month, by volunteers from the Colon Cancer Coalition. Like all Get Your Rear in Gear events, money raised from Nashville's run will help fund screenings and raise awareness about one of the most preventable cancers if it's caught early—and one of the deadliest if it's not.

What frustrates me to no end is that part of the reason colon cancer is the nation's second-leading cancer killer, behind lung cancer, is because people do what I did: attribute their symptoms to something else or assume they're not at risk because it's supposedly an old person's disease. Worse, many doctors also believe this myth, even though incidences of colon cancer have been on the rise among young people for decades.

Regardless, too many in the medical profession hear a young man or woman complain of nausea, fatigue, bloating, and—the most telltale sign of all—blood in his or her bowel movements, and don't order a colonoscopy. And this is because the patient doesn't fit the over-forty-five age profile that ushers in regular colonoscopies and because insurance might not cover it.

As a consequence, colon cancer is ending the lives of people who could easily be saved. All it takes is a simple procedure to either rule out cancer altogether or, in many cases, identify the slow-growing polyps that are the first signs of trouble. And these can be removed right on the table during the procedure.

Sure, a colonoscopy is no picnic. What medical procedure is? But it is a walk in the park compared to the alternative—the alternative that is now my life.

So please, if you are over forty-five, contact your doctor and schedule a colonoscopy today. If you are younger and experiencing symptoms, make an appointment to see your doctor and insist on one. I don't care if you're twenty-five years old. Neither does colon cancer. This disease has no respect for your age, your gender, your healthy lifestyle, or your plans for the future. If it can blindside me, it can blindside you. Please don't let yourself suffer my consequences.

Visit ColonCancerCoalition.org for more information about colon cancer prevention.

• • •

If you are not familiar with cancer, here is a description from the National Cancer Institute. Cancer is the name given to a collection of related diseases. In all types of cancer, some of the body's cells begin to divide without stopping and spread into surrounding tissues. Cancer can start almost anywhere in the human body, which is made up of trillions of cells. Normally, human cells grow and divide to form new cells as the body needs them. When cells grow old or become damaged, they die, and new cells take their place.

When cancer develops, however, this orderly process breaks down. As cells become more and more abnormal, old or damaged cells survive when they should die, and new cells form when they are not needed. These extra cells can divide without stopping and may form growths called tumors. Many cancers form solid tumors, which are masses of tissue. Cancers of the blood, such as leukemia, generally do not form solid tumors. Cancerous tumors are malignant, which means they can spread into, or invade, nearby tissues. In addition, as these tumors grow, some cancer cells can break off and travel to distant places in the body through the blood or the lymph system and form new tumors far from the original tumor.

It has been truly an honor and a privilege to be the vehicle to give voice to these inspiring and heartfelt stories. I am deeply humbled beyond words for the trust these individuals have placed in me to bring their stories to life on these pages. I would like to thank Melissa, Robyn, Helen, Ronn, Jennifer, Bill K., Dana, Bill G., Valerie, Dan, Peggy, Robert, Holly, Nikki, Kim, Gina, Tricia, Debi, Alan, and Kristi for their patience, grace, and courage through the writing and editing process, and their willingness to relive some trauma-charged memories. You are the true heroes for your willingness to be vulnerable and bare all, in an effort to help others. Thank you for reading.

ROBYN'S STORY PART II

———•—●—•———

As my husband and I finished lunch on my forty-sixth birthday, I actually felt a sense of relief that I had heard the results of the tests, as waiting was the hardest for me. I was still mulling over what it meant to have cancer in my lymph nodes, although information felt like power in this moment. This knowledge represented one more step in the direction of feeling in control, defining what would happen next. We celebrated my birthday with the kids on Friday night as I filed away the news of the day, wanting to soak up each moment with my family.

On Monday morning, February 16, my sister and I boarded a plane to Houston, Texas, for my next round of tests at a leading cancer center. My dad lived in Houston, and I was grateful to see him. His comfort was calming to my nerves and filled my heart with a warm loving feeling. My best friend also flew into Houston from Nashville later that evening. I was so thankful to have them all with me, giving me strength and support for the next few days.

We woke up early Tuesday to prepare for the long two days of tests that were scheduled. This leading cancer center approached each test in a very thorough way. We arrived at eight thirty in the morning and checked in at the front desk. As I took each step forward, walking through the halls of this massive hospital, I noticed words of encouragement throughout the building. Knowing that many have fought the battle that I was about to face gave me a sense of hope and helped sustain me. As if I wasn't alone. This was just the beginning of the blessings that God showed me. His love for me was so evident through every step, and while I knew the testing would be grueling, a feeling of peace flooded my veins.

I went back for the first test, which was another mammogram that ended up lasting three hours. The afternoon included more scans—a bone scan, a computerized axial tomography (CAT) scan, a full-body magnetic resonance imaging (MRI) study, and a full-body positron emission photography (PET) scan—each one taking about an hour with waiting in between. About six thirty, the nurse announced we were finished for the day and to come back the next morning at eight thirty. While I was exhausted from the grueling day, and my chest hurt a little from the three-hour mammogram, knowing that these actions were leading us one step closer to more information gave me energy. We arrived the next day for more tests. This time we started with lab work, followed by several different kinds of biopsies. A physician who spoke with a French accent was leading the biopsy efforts. He was determined to take his time and be thorough in his process, which I appreciated. While it was long and arduous, I was very grateful that he found the nodes in my chest that were of concern. The toughest test of all was the one that required me to drink red liquid—as I drank it, every cell in my body felt like it was on fire, like I was in a sauna, from the tips of my toes to the top of my head.

At the end of the two days of testing, we met with the lead oncologist for my case. My sister and best friend held my hands as we listened to all the details of the testing results. He confirmed the diagnosis of triple negative breast cancer. My heart sank with the news, as if it was the first time I had heard those words. I was really grateful that my sister wrote down everything the doctor said so I could reflect on the information later. When I had heard the diagnosis the first time, I found myself having a hard time remembering the details, due to the stressful nature of the conversation. Having my loved ones present and taking notes helped me to process later, comparing the details we each heard.

We left the cancer center and returned to my dad's house, exhausted and sad with the reality I was facing. We flew home to our respective cities the next morning. As soon as we arrived back in Denver, I called an oncologist who had come highly recommended to me from a friend. I felt divinely guided to this physician and knew how important it was for me to get one more opinion, given that I did not feel comfortable with the first physician we met with in Denver. Once my husband and I met him a few days later, we both were confident that he was the right physician for me. He was kind and nurturing, with a humble presence, and he was willing to spend time explaining all the results in an easy-to-understand way. When he finished walking us through all of the results, he stood there and paused. Something didn't feel quite right with my diagnosis to him. He studied the information and then looked up at us. He said, "Robyn, there is something that is not quite adding up to me. I want to be very certain and ensure we have an accurate diagnosis for you, as it will dictate the treatment path. I am going to send your lab work to a laboratory in California. It's hard to know exactly how long it will take to get the results, so plan on a few weeks. I will be in touch soon."

We said good-bye, and my husband and I walked to the car, hand in hand. He looked at me and said, "I know the waiting will be hard. I will be right here by your side, whatever you need. I am so grateful for your doctor and his determination and thoroughness in getting another opinion. I love you." We hugged for a while when we reached the car. Having his unconditional support enabled me to be calm in the midst of the fear, knowing I was not alone.

One of the things on my bucket list was going to New York City to see *The Tonight Show with Jimmy Fallon*. Four of my close friends and I were able to get last-minute seats for the show, a week after my appointment. What an amazing experience and great time we had together! We laughed out loud many times, and the laughing helped calm my nerves a little, although I still felt anxious knowing what was to come. It was also very hard to be away from my husband. He had decided to stay home with the kids and wanted me to experience this show with my friends. I knew I needed him more than ever. Another great trip I took was with my sister, as she wanted to help me achieve another bucket list item. We flew to Los Angeles to watch *The Ellen DeGeneres Show*. What a memorable experience it was! We took long walks on the beach, taking in the breathtaking view as the waves crashed against the shore. We also enjoyed a little retail therapy and ate some mouth-watering food.

After I had filled several weeks with trips that created memorable experiences, my doctor's office finally called and scheduled an appointment to discuss the results. The night before I saw the doctor, I tossed and turned in bed as fear started to gain a foothold in my thoughts. I was most afraid of the type of treatment I would need to endure. *Will I have to go through chemotherapy?* I wondered, holding out hope that just maybe I wouldn't have to. Then images filled my mind of what I would look like going through chemotherapy: throwing up often and losing my hair, looking like a cancer patient, wearing scarves to hide my baldness. The exhaustion took over, and I finally dozed off to sleep. My husband woke me the next morning, reminding me that the time for answers was finally here.

As my husband drove us to the appointment, a vivid memory came back to me from a few months prior. There I was, standing in my friend's living room with my Bible study group, a group of seven women. It was quiet for a minute, and I heard God speak to me. He said, "One of you is going to get cancer." I was startled and looked around, realizing that I was the only one who had heard those words. As I reflected on that time now, I became cognizant of a symptom I had been experiencing but had discounted. I would watch a car drive by, and it would move in frames, like slow motion.

I willed myself to ignore it. *It's nothing* I thought. I made a mental note to ask my doctor about this symptom.

My husband and I walked into the exam room, holding hands, feeling a sense of relief that we would have the correct diagnosis shortly. My doctor came in and said, "Well, Robyn, so it looks like you do not have triple negative breast cancer after all. Your type of cancer is called HER2-positive. And the number of HER2 cells you have is more than I have ever seen, twenty-seven, and normal is six." My husband and I looked at each other, in part worried at the number of cells and in part feeling so grateful for this doctor and his willingness to keep looking until he had all the answers. I then decided to ask him if the problem with my eyes was related to the cancer. He said, "Yes, that is an early sign of cancer when your eyes see in frames rather than fluid motion." *Wow,* I thought, *and I discounted that symptom.* Given the way the events unfolded, we knew God had a hand in leading us to this doctor and guiding him to look further. Having the right treatment plan with the right drugs was critically important to enabling my highest chance of survival. He said I needed eighteen weeks of chemotherapy to start, and there was 65 percent chance that the cancer would be eliminated when I was finished. Because my cancer was so fast growing, I started with chemotherapy, endured radiation, and had a double mastectomy followed by reconstructive surgery. I closed my eyes as I processed the word *chemotherapy*, taking in the magnitude of what we had just learned and the difference my doctor was making in my life.

Treatment Experience

As I worked through preparing myself, spiritually, mentally, physically, and emotionally, for the treatment, I felt so much gratitude, thinking about all the people I had at my side, providing support and reminding me that I was strong and ready to face the treatments. I knew that in each moment, the only way I was really going to have the strength to get through this was to completely surrender all my fears and lay them down. God showed up over and over again, from leading me to the right doctor, to having such supportive family and friends, and for putting people who encouraged me in my path.

I had a physician who had proved to me that he had a vested interest in giving me the highest chance of survival, building such trust with me that I could let go and follow his recommended protocol. He became my biggest cheerleader during the treatment, boosting my ability to endure day in and day out. In addition, my husband and sister went to every appointment with me. My doctor ordered six rounds of a drug regimen that included Carboplatin, Taxol, Herceptin, and Perjeta, every twenty-one days. I would go in the day after my infusion to get a shot of Neulasta to help build my immune system. And at times when I felt extremely ill, I would go in for an infusion of fluid the following Monday.

The doctor's office assigned a navigator to guide the scheduling of the many tests, to provide reminders of the actions I needed to take, and to inform me of any changes. As a cancer patient, I now had a cadre of doctors who worked together on my case, including a primary care physician, an ob-gyn, a surgeon, a radiation oncologist, a medical oncologist, and a plastic surgeon. Having a navigator made it possible for me to keep it all straight.

I showed up for my first infusion on March 12, 2015, with my husband and my sister by my side. The first round was somewhat smooth, and I didn't feel any different at first. I went for a walk the next day and had energy. Two days later, I felt nauseous and unsettled. My physician told me that it was highly likely my hair would start falling out, given the drugs I was taking. I didn't really believe him, thinking inside that I was going to have a different experience and would be able to keep my hair. After eighteen days, I ran my fingers through my hair and felt what I feared most—my hair falling out into my hands. I closed my eyes and felt this deep vulnerability permeate my veins in a way I had never felt before. I knew I had no control, as this first physically noticeable change in my new state of being a cancer patient emerged. I knew it would draw attention to me, something I was not used to. I said a prayer for God to fill me with peace and give me strength to endure this humbling experience.

And then an idea popped in my head: *I will just shave my head, take control over the situation, and drive my reaction to this side effect.* Yes! I called my family and close friends and invited them over for a big shave-your-head party. I was grateful to have everyone around me in the comfort of my home. I had long hair at the time, and my hairdressers started the process by making some fun, sassy, short-lived cuts. I pranced around the room taking in my new sassy look. Then they shaved my head. The feeling of shaving my head was very freeing. My sweet cousin surprised me and showed up, traveling all the way from Arkansas. He ended up only staying an hour, which was so amazing to me. So kind, that he would make the effort to see me. Later that day, a friend of mine completely shocked me by shaving her own head, and there she was just like me. I have to say that being bald was the hardest part of my cancer experience. Over time, being bald allowed me to realize that my identity was not based on what I looked like, but who I was inside, fighting to survive. After all, I believed my hair would grow back.

On day twenty-one, I went in for my second infusion. Almost immediately after the drugs started penetrating my blood, I had an allergic reaction. I started shivering and shaking, and my heart-beat became irregular. I began taking deep belly breaths to try to calm down as four nurses descended on me, checking things out. My husband was looking at me with deep concern, and my sister started crying. My friend looked at me with a calming face, as she had fought cancer ten years earlier. She had a sense of peace and helped me in so many ways throughout my journey. She kept saying, "You can do this. You're okay, just breathe." The nurse gave me some Pepcid and Benadryl, which helped calm the shaking and shivering and made my heartbeat a little more normal. The nurses moved me into the closed-door room adjacent to the infusion area to monitor me closely. This reaction changed my course of treatment from then on. Because of the way I responded, I would always go in this room to get my infusions. I would lie down, and the infusions would take twice as long, but it minimized the chance that I would experience a negative reaction.

Each infusion I endured made me sicker inside as I felt the medicine run through my veins. The accumulation of the drugs was debilitating. I would lie there as the drugs pumped into my body, feeling like each cell was being depleted of oxygen. My fists were always clenched tightly like I was fighting a war against the drugs. It was like an electrical current driving through my spine and shrinking my cells. As I lay there on the bed, I needed to be quiet to handle these feelings. I wasn't able to focus on TV or read a book. I would doze off to sleep sometimes during the infusion from pure exhaustion. I would pray and ask God to get me through each moment. I knew that He would give me the strength that I needed. His presence allowed me to rest. After day ten, I began to regain my strength. I was able to take walks, and my appetite would slowly start to come back. I always had my chemotherapy infusions on a Thursday, and two days later the sickness would kick in. I realized that if I went in for hydration the day after my infusion, it would take the edge off. The sickness lasted for about ten solid days, and then I would feel like I had some energy to get up and go do something. I also experienced a couple of bacterial infections on my head. Each time was gut-wrenchingly painful. The nurse gave me antibiotics to help heal the infections. The nurses were so humble and compassionate, always focusing on my every need with such caring hearts.

I met amazing people through my treatment. Something I learned when I showed up for the first time was how comfortable I felt with complete strangers, knowing we each were connected by a common diagnosis, cancer. We formed a group and called ourselves "Chemo Warriors." One woman had stage IV cancer in her spine and breast at the time and today is in remission. I will never forget looking at her as we were both having our ports connected. She told me the doctors had given her two years to live. Throughout our time together in treatments, we prayed together and refused to accept that pronouncement. And another friend, Nikki, who is featured later in this book, was enduring cancer treatment for the second time. She is one of the strongest women I know. The encouragement she gave me was so helpful. I met another dear friend, a man who drives a Harley. He wore chaps on the first day I met him and had a long gray ponytail. He was an amazing witness of faith and kindness, and we are still great friends today. And Jennifer, a strong warrior with stage III breast cancer, who is also featured in this book, was such a positive encouragement.

When the chemotherapy was finished, I started radiation, which lasted for six weeks. It was five days a week, and I was in and out within five minutes. One thing that I was never told was how the effects of radiation would stay with me. Physical therapy and massage were critical to surviving the side effects, and keeping my skin well hydrated with lotion was crucial as my skin burned.

There is nothing that could have really prepared me for the surgery I had, called a double mastectomy. My breast surgeon was a breast cancer survivor, which gave me a sense of hope. I chose to have my reconstruction as soon after as was feasible. The most important thing for surviving such a complicated procedure was to stay ahead of the pain, which I did with pain management therapy. The plastic surgeon placed expanders in my body with drains to allow my skin to stretch to hold space for the implants. Once my body healed, the expanders were removed, and the breast implants were placed in my chest with more drains. The drains helped to make sure I didn't get an infection and were removed once my body stopped producing blood. It took a good six weeks before I was able to resume light activity.

Our kids managed to navigate the changes in our family as I endured the treatments. We kept their schedules full and made sure they were surrounded by family and friends. My husband had a lot on his plate in caring for me and looking after the kids when I was in the trenches of my illness. My parents lived out of town, but their love and support were always present. My husband's parents and brothers, and my sister and her husband were always there to help us. My friends rallied in such beautiful ways, such as bringing us food, stopping by to say hi, praying for me, and reaching out via text. I received flowers almost every day throughout my treatments from different friends and family members, which I cherished. I also took advantage of a service that would come clean my house once a week for free, for a few months. In addition, I spoke to several women who had walked through cancer before me, which helped me to compare things I was hearing and know what to expect physically.

Nothing could have prepared me to hear the words, "You have cancer." I felt a definite shift in my spirit. Suddenly, all the first world problems in my life became very small. I wasn't fearful, but I felt complete disbelief. I would never have guessed this journey would be a chapter in my life. And in some ways, I'm thankful for it. I grew through the challenging treatment, and it deepened my faith.

It has been three and a half years now, and I still see my oncologist every six months. I always breathe a sigh of relief after I receive my blood results and know I have "no evidence of disease," a term used in medicine to represent no sign of cancer. I have realized how important it is to be more present in each moment. The mind, body, and spirit are so connected. I learned how important my diet is to my health, as everything I put into my body now really does matter. I used to internalize a lot of my emotions; I would shut down and hold onto anger or sadness. I have learned that it truly contributes to illness. I found freedom in my faith and in knowing that I no longer had to carry burdens by myself. I also learned that, as long as I have my health, I can truly handle anything that life throws at me. This experience truly changed my outlook on death and I no longer have a fear of dying. Chemotherapy was so hard on my body that I knew I had to completely rely on the Lord to bring me through each breath at times. Cancer was a season in my life in which I learned valuable lessons, although I would never wish for anyone to have to endure this horrible disease.

Advice for Others

How I supported myself

- Trusting and believing that God had me; sometimes it was minute by minute, but I never gave up hope.
- Praying, listening to music, laughing, spending time in the fresh air, eating healthy, walking when I could.

How others supported me

- I made sure someone was with me at each appointment; my sister would take notes for me, and we would discuss what we each heard afterward.
- I accepted offers of help around the house; people made grocery runs, brought over meals and drinks, cleaned our home, did loads of laundry, ran errands, and shuttled my children to and from school.
- Someone made a blanket for me that represented breast cancer; it brought me comfort when I slept.
- Friends sent flowers weekly for several months.
- Friends stopped by, allowing me to feel connected to some normalcy; they also mailed cards, sent me encouraging texts, and brought thoughtful gifts.
- The church provided a meal train for six months, which was so helpful for my husband and my children; my food aversion was very strong.

Helpful tips

- If you know someone experiencing a cancer diagnosis, know that the family also needs support and a safe place to process their emotions.
- Stay up to date on preventive health screenings and seek help if you are experience any symptoms.

Surprising experiences

I was at the salon getting a manicure and pedicure one day. A woman walked up to me, as if she was on a mission and was very clear about her goal. She said, "I am twenty years out. You can do this," and then proceeded to pay for my services.

I was at dinner one night in Minneapolis, Minnesota, after I had just finished my last chemotherapy infusion. I was in the middle of conversation with my friends when I noticed a woman walking toward our table. She said, "I figure that you are a cancer patient, and I am also. I just want you to know that you can do this." Then she walked away, never to be seen again.

One day, my warrior group was at one of our houses having lunch. All of a sudden, we heard the doorbell ring. We were not expecting anyone. We opened the door and found a woman, Kim, standing there, looking determined. She said, "Am I at the right place?" She looked the same as us—we all were bald, which we giggled about. She continued, "I am a cancer survivor. I am here to pray with all of you." After she finished praying, she took some oil out of her purse and anointed each of us, saying a prayer with such compassion. That was so impactful to me. She had driven over an hour to reach us.

HELEN'S STORY

———•———

It was about six thirty Monday morning on April 8, 2013. I was taking a shower and preparing to go to work. It felt like a normal Monday, although thoughts of the exciting events coming up were racing through my mind. My youngest child would graduate from Vanderbilt University in a few weeks, and we had planned a family vacation to Germany right after graduation. With my youngest graduating from college, I was imagining what life would be like with both of my children out in the working world, a time in life marking the end of a parenting era. Memories of my daughter as a baby flooded my mind as I considered this next phase of life. I was feeling a little anxious about the transition, although I knew she was well prepared. She was strong-willed and independent, and had already accepted a job in Atlanta, Georgia. I was fifty-five years old at the time.

As I showered, I shifted my focus to complete a breast self-exam, something I had become diligent about doing monthly following my mother and grandmother's breast cancer diagnoses. I was avid about getting my annual mammograms as well and had just had one four months before. As I raised my left arm and felt around, my fingers brushed over something foreign—a lump about the size of a pea, hard to the touch, although not visible to the eye.

My heart started beating rapidly, and I felt lightheaded, as I put my right hand on the shower wall to steady my balance. *Oh no, what could this be, another benign tumor or something worse?* I wondered as I tried to catch my breath. Finding a lump was something I had experienced before—in 1995 right after my mother was diagnosed. I had been through the process of a biopsy, learned it was benign, and had the lump removed. As a result, I already had a relationship with a surgeon, something that was very helpful in getting appointments scheduled in a reasonable amount of time. I had learned at this point in my life that I had fibrocystic breast tissue and had since grown accustomed to the rope-like feeling of the tissue when I did breast self-exams. As I stood there a little paralyzed in the shower, water pulsing down on my head, it felt like the drops of water were moving in slow motion, and I lost track of what I was doing. A few minutes later, I gathered my composure and finished my shower.

I toweled off and put on my robe. My heart was still racing as I went to find my phone. I dialed my husband's number, as he had already left for work. When I heard his voice on the other end, I said, "Honey, I found a lump in my breast just now while I was showering. I'm going to call my doctor as soon as the office opens. I'm a little freaked out. I'll keep you posted." My husband was supportive and reassured me that he was there for me, whatever I needed. Feeling his comfort calmed me down a little, gave me strength to push through, and helped quiet the chaos in my mind. I wondered as I drove if this would be a more impactful life change shaping up, more impactful than both of my children being out of school for the first time. I could feel my stomach turn over as I continued to process what I had just discovered. I didn't know what it was exactly, and not knowing made me feel a little scattered and distracted. I kept looking at my watch every few minutes, wondering if the doctor's office was open yet. I arrived at my company's office building, parked, and went inside, not really speaking to anyone I passed along the way. I glanced at my watch, and it was finally time to call.

I reached my doctor's nurse and explained what I had discovered. "Is it best for me to come in for a visit as the next step?" I asked. Given my family history of breast cancer, the nurse recommended I call the surgeon first. I thanked her and hung up. I could see the emails filling up my inbox on the computer screen out of the corner of my eye, although they seemed far away in my priorities in this moment.

I took a deep breath, dialed the surgeon's office, and explained my situation to his scheduler. She said, "Oh yes, Helen, I see your record in the computer. It turns out he has had a cancellation; would you be able to come in tomorrow morning?"

I replied quickly, "Oh yes, thank you, I'll be there. Good-bye." I called my husband to let him know and then tried to focus on work. All of a sudden, the mounting emails felt different to me, much less important than the discovery I was still processing from a few hours before. I tried to keep myself busy, taking care of business and going to meetings. My mind kept shifting back to the shower, not knowing whether this was something to worry about. My business partners noticed a difference in my demeanor—my responses were short, and I seemed on edge. I could feel each of them giving me puzzled looks. I decided to tell them what I had found, as I knew I would be out the next day, although uncertain for how long. They were both supportive and asked how they could help. We discussed a project that needed some attention while I was going to be away, and one of my partners agreed to cover for me.

That evening, I found myself snapping at my husband over dinner for no reason. I went to sleep early, exhausted from the mind gymnastics of the day. The next day, my husband went with me to the appointment. The surgeon recommended a biopsy as a next step so we could learn more. He left the room and returned with good news—he would be able to do the biopsy in about thirty minutes. A needle biopsy was fairly standard as a next step to determine whether the mass was something to worry about. I went out in the waiting room, tried to distract myself with reading a magazine, and then started pacing the floor. My mind would not focus on any one thing at a time, just the chaotic thoughts of what this mass could be and what would happen next. The nurse called me back for the biopsy, and my husband came back with me. I lay there watching the doctor's face and the screen as he started the biopsy. The mass was pretty deep in my left breast. He tried one approach, then another, although he was unable to reach the mass due to the location. He stopped and looked at me and said, "Helen, we are going to have to schedule a more in-depth biopsy due to the location. I am not going to be able to use the needle biopsy after all. We will get it scheduled as fast as possible." His response seemed to make sense to me, so I got dressed and went out to the front desk. The clerk had already been able to schedule a more in-depth biopsy for that Friday, just a few days away, called a core biopsy.

I was grateful to leave the office with a next step on the schedule. I knew distractions would be helpful, so I attempted to keep as busy as possible and continued with my normal daily activities. I went home instead of back to the office and let my partners know. I didn't want to worry anyone and decided to keep this discovery to myself, my husband, and my business partners until we knew more. I kept my appointment with my trainer the next morning, Wednesday, and ran on the treadmill on Thursday, maintaining my normal routine and hoping that exercise would give my chaotic mind a break.

I was able to distract myself with work and exercise until Friday finally arrived. My husband went with me to the appointment. I undressed and hoisted myself up onto the table. The doctor numbed the area and started the procedure. I watched her as she continued, glancing back at the screen and then at her face. While she didn't say anything to me, I could tell by the way she was looking at the screen that something was wrong, probably more than just a benign tumor. She finished the procedure and let me know that I would get a call early the next week with more information. While I was somewhat relieved that this step in the process was complete, I knew waiting over the weekend would be difficult, and my chaotic mind would continue to race forward: *What if this is cancer, what will happen next?* The waiting felt similar to slogging through deep mud; everything was moving in slow motion after that.

Wanting to keep my normal routine and distract myself as much as possible, I kept my plans to walk the 5.8-mile loop in Percy Warner Park the next morning with my girlfriends. I decided to keep my discovery to myself and focused on listening to their stories, although my mind would wander back to this mass and whether it was cancer growing in my body. It felt comforting to be surrounded by good friends and be out in nature in my favorite park. As I said good-bye and headed home, my mind shifted back to this mass growing inside of me. I thought about my grandmother, who had been diagnosed with breast cancer at age sixty-two. Then my mother popped into my head. She had survived inflammatory stage IV breast cancer when I was thirty-seven. She was fifty-eight at the time, in 1995, and had been told she had only a 10 percent chance of surviving.

Instead of feeling helpless, my mother took charge of her situation and approached her cancer treatment with thoughtful planning, diligence, and organization. She was determined to survive, despite the odds. During her treatment, which included high-dose chemotherapy and a bone marrow transplant, my mom's immune system was so compromised that they put her in isolation in the hospital for twenty-two days. Despite the outward appearance of a bleak outcome, my mother pushed through, doing all she could to focus her mind on healing. She practiced creative visualization, including imagining a Pac-Man like creature from the 1980s video game eating the cancer cells, one by one. As I thought of her experience, I was able to relax a little. She had modeled warrior behavior for me and succeeded in beating her cancer. *If she could do it,* I thought, *so can I, if I have cancer.* As I processed this memory, I recalled that my mother was in good health and still going strong at seventy-five. Yes, that could be me also. I was able to keep busy with distractions and made it through the weekend.

I walked into my company's office building on Monday morning, put my things in my office, and headed to the conference room for our leadership meeting. I kept looking at my phone as I walked, wondering when the call would come with results. When I sat down in the conference room chair, I decided to leave my phone out on the table next to my notebook. While I was present in person, my mind kept wandering off to thinking about this mass and whether it was cancer. All of a sudden, my phone lit up, and I knew it was the surgeon. I excused myself and stepped out of the room. One of my partners saw the worry on my face and followed me outside. She stood next to me as I listened to the results, hearing the bone-crushing words that it was cancer and what would happen next. I hung up, and she wrapped her arms around me. A feeling of shock filled my body as the words 'you have cancer' settled into my soul.

I wanted to get to my office quickly, given this news, not wanting anyone to see me as the words replayed in my mind. I walked down the hall and closed my office door behind me as my business partner called my husband, who worked in a building that was three doors down. He stopped what he was doing and rushed over quickly. He walked through my office doorway and reached out to put his arms around me. As I felt the comfort of his arms around me, the weight of the news hit me hard. I let go and started sobbing uncontrollably for what felt like ten minutes. I pulled away and looked in his eyes as if it were the first time, taking in the details of his face. He said, "Honey, we are going to get through this, I will be at your side every step of the way. Do you think we should call the children and tell them? And what time is the appointment with the surgeon this afternoon?" We discussed the details and made a plan to call our daughter now and wait until our son got off work to tell him.

I knew my daughter would take this news differently than my son, knowing that an element of her reaction would be wondering about her own mortality and the chances of her getting breast cancer. I took a deep breath and we called her together, on speaker phone. "Hi honey, we have some tough news to share with you. I found a lump in my breast and just learned it is cancer. We are going to the surgeon's office this afternoon; would you like to join us? We really don't know anything else right now." There was silence on the other end of the line for a few seconds. When she spoke, I could hear her voice become shaky as she asked a few more questions. She definitely wanted to go with me to the surgeon's appointment. As we hung up, my concern grew not only for me, but for how my daughter was processing this news.

My husband, my daughter, and I went to the surgeon's office that afternoon. The surgeon looked at me as my husband held my hand and said, "Helen, it is cancer, although we don't yet know much more. We need to wait for more detailed biopsy reports. We caught it early, although it's important to be aggressive in starting treatment quickly." He paused for a minute as he took in the weight of his words and my reaction. Then he said, "I know this is a lot of information and probably hard to swallow. Do you have any questions for me?" My brain shut down at that point as my heart started pounding, my face turned a dark pink, and my stomach became nauseous. Fear was spreading through my body. While the surgeon had tried to reassure me that we'd caught it early, I struggled to keep my composure, knowing my family history and the odds that I would need chemotherapy. We thanked the surgeon and left the office.

The waiting was crippling my ability to function and keep a clear head. I wasn't sure when I would know what type of cancer I had so I could move forward with a plan. My doctor called on Wednesday to provide more information. He said, "Helen, your cancer is not a hormonal type, meaning the type of cancer that has receptors for estrogen or progesterone and is fed by hormones. It is one of the two types of breast cancer that are not hormone fed, what's called HER2 and triple negative, stage II. We do need to move quickly here, as this type of cancer is very aggressive and tough to treat." As he finished explaining the details, my mind raced forward, starting to imagine the worst, as this didn't sound good. I knew now I was up for a fight to beat this and would need an oncologist quickly. It wasn't until two days later that I learned my type of cancer was triple negative. I was scared to death, although somewhat relieved to have answers and be able to build a treatment plan.

Now was the time to let others know and to find a good oncologist. I called my friend, who had survived breast cancer, to get her advice. I let my business partners know what we had learned. Determining what would happen next in this process of my new diagnosis while I was also planning for my daughter's graduation was completely overwhelming. I fell into bed, feeling exhausted and out of touch with my body. The next morning, I started making calls, although none of them led to an appointment. I tried a couple of approaches without any luck. Through each conversation, I was beginning to learn how important it was to be an advocate for myself, to leverage the relationships I had, and to be aggressive in getting the appointment scheduled. I called a few friends and was able to secure an appointment with an oncologist, who had been my mother's doctor and a friend's doctor. I had remembered his no-nonsense attitude and appreciated that he was a straight shooter.

My husband and I arrived at the appointment the following week, on April 23, with lots of questions. I wanted all the information I could gather, feeling that if I knew, I would be in control. Hearing the words that I had cancer was one of the most helpless feelings I had ever experienced, as I was used to being in control of my life. I started asking him question after question, and then he stopped me. He looked me in the eye and said, "Actually, Helen, it would be good for you to chill on all the questions, as we don't know very much. Here is where you need to focus. Having surgery of some type is the only way for us to determine if the cancer has spread to your lymph nodes. We really need to know this before figuring out a treatment plan. I think you may know your type of cancer is triple negative." My mind was swirling with all this information and the potential decisions I needed to make next. As I sat with his words, I trusted his guidance and believed that my next step was to focus on getting through the surgery, not trying to jump ahead. We discussed the options of having a lumpectomy or a mastectomy. Given the timing of my daughter's graduation and my keen interest in attending, I chose a lumpectomy to remove the tumor and test the lymph nodes. The doctor said, "Okay, then let's get the lumpectomy scheduled as quickly as possible. I recommend you undergo chemotherapy after the lumpectomy due to the fast-growing type of cancer." I knew that I could always go back and have a mastectomy if needed and attending my daughter's graduation at this point was my priority. As I walked out to the front desk, I learned that my lumpectomy had been scheduled for Monday, April 29.

In my effort to maintain my normal routine, I decided to keep my plans to participate in the Rock and Roll half marathon on April 27, the weekend before my procedure, with two of my walking buddies. It helped me focus on something other than my diagnosis or my daughter's upcoming graduation, both situations that felt overwhelming to me. I was grateful to have friends supporting my effort to keep a normal routine, despite the diagnosis that hung over my head. I had completed several half marathons before in mild weather, although this one was memorable, one of those races with driving rain throughout the 13.1-mile course. We supported each other through each mile and somehow made it to the finish line, where my husband was waiting for me. Seeing him filled my heart with joy and gave me peace amid the uncertainty of what would happen next. As I think back to that moment when I learned I had cancer, I recall seeing a difference in his actions from that day forward. He shifted into protective mode, wanting to be at my side every step of the way. It fascinated me to see him change. He no longer wanted to travel for work but wanted to be near me in case I needed something. As I sat and reflected on his unconditional love, I realize now that the longest period of time we had gone without being apart in our thirty-five years of marriage was during my cancer treatment—when I finally made him travel for an important business meeting.

Treatment Experience

The time period of waiting from diagnosis to treatment plan was filled with worry and wonder. *What kind of chemotherapy would I need? Would I lose my hair? What would happen next in the process?* I am a planner by nature, so the fear of the unknown was percolating in my mind and would make itself known when I least expected it. I felt paralyzed and in an uncomfortable state of ambiguity. Once I had a plan, I felt like I could move forward with my life.

I showed up the morning of April 29 for my lumpectomy, with my husband by my side. They also planned to insert a port-a-cath for chemotherapy during the procedure. The tumor was situated way up under my arm on the left side, which was a challenging position to navigate with all the nerves and blood vessels. I was grateful to have been sedated, as the procedure felt very painful. My daughter's graduation was still a week away, so I had time to recover. The surgeon said not to lift anything and that I would be sore for a few weeks. Somehow, I wanted to believe he was wrong. It was just a lumpectomy; it couldn't be that hard to recover from. Boy, I was wrong! I struggled to raise my left arm for weeks after the procedure.

My husband and I showed up to my follow-up appointment with the oncologist once he had the results from the lumpectomy. He said, "The good news is no cancer is showing up in your lymph nodes from what we can tell. While there is no standard drug regimen for your type of cancer, there are two drugs I would recommend using together that have shown promising results. I want to give you the highest chance of survival." He went on to tell me that he couldn't guarantee anything. I really appreciated his honesty in admitting he couldn't know for sure what the outcome would be. I thought about all he had said, looked at him in the eye, and said, "I think I want to get a second opinion."

He replied, "Yes, I think you should. A second opinion is a good idea." I left his office with confidence that while I was facing a difficult road, I could trust this person to guide the steps along the path if I chose him as my doctor.

I made an appointment for a second opinion within a few days. My goal was to be open to this doctor's recommendation. He validated the approach of having a lumpectomy first, which was helpful. He recommended a different drug regimen, one that had much tougher side effects. What I really wanted was for someone to tell me, "We've got this. This is what you need to do." Since there was no standard protocol, I wasn't going to hear that. I thought about the two options and decided to go with my mother's oncologist, the first doctor I met with. I trusted him. I knew I could always try the other drug regimen if the first one didn't work.

Following the lumpectomy procedure, I was not able to lift anything or start chemotherapy for thirty days. The waiting was so tough; I just wanted to move forward on the plan. Since I had to wait anyway, we decided to go on our trip to Germany after my daughter's graduation. I was still sore and couldn't lift anything while we were traveling. I was quite a sight for strangers, as I looked like a queen or a lady of leisure, waiting around for my husband and daughter to carry my luggage. I remember getting strange looks from women near us, although I felt completely spoiled. After all, I appeared perfectly normal, and there were no visible signs of recent surgery. We rode trains and subways everywhere and really enjoyed seeing the country. The trip was a welcome distraction from my diagnosis as we created lasting memories together. It felt like God-given timing to have been able to get away and not focus on what would happen next, and a helpful respite from the mental gymnastics going on in my mind.

When we returned, I started my six rounds of chemotherapy infusions with Taxotere and Carboplatin. I went once every three weeks, providing enough time in between for my body to recover. I experienced every side effect I have ever heard of during chemo: nausea, change in taste buds, neuropathy, mouth sores, thrush, lost hair, and a messed-up colon. During the three-week cycle, I felt the worst during the first week and gained more strength each subsequent week. I figured out that days three and four were the hardest days for symptoms, so I isolated myself during those days. I put my hands in frozen gloves during the infusions so I would not lose my nails and ate ice chips for the duration. I learned how to manage the symptoms in a proactive way and had some helpful medicine to ease the pain. I ignored the mouth sores after the first infusion, and then learned the hard way that I needed to speak up. I was not able to tolerate eating anything acidic, such as tomatoes, and had to stop drinking my hot lemon water in the morning. My stomach could still handle coffee and wine, although both tasted disgusting to me. I figured out that if I ate small meals, my stomach was able to digest the food easier. I was hyper-focused on nutrition, trying to figure out anything I could do to lessen the symptoms. One drink I was able to tolerate was green tea, which I consumed several times a day. I am not able to drink green tea to this day, as it reminds me of chemotherapy. Someone had told me that I might get neuropathy and what to do if it happened, which was really helpful.

Following chemotherapy, I followed up with my oncologist about the next steps. We discussed whether having a mastectomy or going through radiation treatment would give me a higher chance of survival. He said the outcomes were better for people who underwent radiation. We discussed the pros and cons, and I chose seven weeks of radiation treatment, every day for five days, finishing the day before Thanksgiving. The only side effect of radiation was extreme tiredness. Compared to the chemotherapy, I was grateful that the side effects were minimal. I decided against having a mastectomy.

Despite my husband's devoted nature and tending to my every need, I was not always kind and loving towards him. The chemicals running through my veins had extreme effects on my brain and my body. At one point, when we had finished eating and he was trying to help by putting away food, I yelled at him and said I was going to divorce him, as he was using the wrong size Tupperware container. I was grateful for his compassion and willingness to stay by my side, withstanding my emotional outbursts.

I approached my cancer treatment like a project, similar to the way my mother had. My two coaches, personal friends who were cancer survivors, told me to walk every day, even during chemotherapy and radiation. "It will help you so much," they said, "and enable you to heal quicker. It will also help you mentally. Even when you feel terrible, like your guts are pouring out of your body, it's important to change your view, get outside to walk, and keep your body moving, enable your brain to reset." These words permeated my being every day and gave me strength to get outside, even if to walk only ten steps.

When all active treatment was done, I faced the toughest part of my cancer experience. During the treatment process, I was checking off each step in my plan, leading me to feel like I was in control of something, if only to complete a task. My oncologist told me that there was nothing else I could do to lower the risk of recurrence. It was so hard to not feel like I was actively fighting it. I was bald and exhausted, and people were saying, "You're done with treatment!" I did not feel done. I found myself getting mad and yelling at people who were trying to be supportive, as they thought I was finished. Although active treatment was behind me, I was still feeling the effects of the chemotherapy on how my brain processed information, and knew I needed to be vigilant for five years as the risk of recurrence was high. I honestly didn't ever feel done. I would hear, "Aren't you so excited, you're finished!" These types of statements did not sit well with me. I had no idea what the next five years would bring. After all, I could not have predicted this diagnosis. I decided to join a cancer support group at a place called Gilda's Club, a cancer support organization dedicated to providing encouragement, education, and hope to all people impacted by cancer. It was in those moments, the sessions with other cancer patients, when I felt most validated and most normal. Some people in the group had finished treatment, while others were going through it. I made the decision in that moment that cancer would not define me. It was just a season in my life, not who I was.

Following the end of my treatment, I was instructed to visit my doctor every three months for five years. He had shared with me that the chances of recurrence would drop significantly after five years. Whenever I prepared to go back for a visit, I would grow irritable and short with people around me, as fear would permeate my mind. By the time my birthday came on May 15, I would have the results and be able to breathe a sigh of relief that another year had passed. May 15 became my marker in my mind every year for survival. I turned sixty in 2018, and that was my five-year mark.

One of the ways this cancer experience has changed me is in how I support others. Now, no matter what is going on in my life, when someone calls and asks for help, I drop what I am doing and show up. I keep cards in my desk and mail them out to let friends know I am thinking of them. The experience has also reshaped how I think about my own life and whether tomorrow will come. I know now I am not invincible and recognize how important appreciating each day is. I learned flexibility and patience early in my son's life, as he was born with a series of birth defects that required twenty-eight surgeries and numerous treatments as he grew up, many in the first five years of his life. He is thriving today, which brings me great joy.

One final thing I want to share about the cancer experience is the long-lasting effect of the chemotherapy drugs and radiation. My doctor recommended that I not make any big life decisions for at least a year after my treatment. The drugs are designed to eradicate the cancer cells, and in the process, also deplete healthy cells, causing longer-term side effects. My ability to process information quickly and think strategically in a planning session with clients was heavily diminished after chemotherapy. It took two full years before I was able to facilitate strategic planning sessions again and three full years before my brain would accurately process numbers. In addition, lymphedema, swelling in my left arm, set in two years after treatment. Lymphedema is caused by a blockage in the lymphatic system. There is no cure, and it needs to be proactively managed to keep it from getting worse. I now wear a compression garment on my hand, arm, and torso during the day and different compression garments every night. While all of these impacts to my daily life are difficult to accept, I am grateful to have survived and have learned to live with them.

Advice for Others

How I supported myself
- I learned how to ask for help, something I had not been good at before.
- I shared my journey on a website called CaringBridge and posted every three weeks—it was a helpful way to communicate, and it was therapeutic; I received thousands of messages of support and would read and reread them before my chemo infusions.
- I would go into work some days to get my mind off the season I was in and find something helpful to distract me from where I was, reminding me of the temporary nature of my current season in life.
- I developed a project plan to manage the details and logged my symptoms; I was able to look back and see trends on what was working or not, which was extremely helpful and enabled me to feel like I had some kind of control.

- I taught myself to take deep belly breaths and learned how to meditate.
- I was obnoxious about staying away from germs and would not shake hands or hug people.
- I figured out through trial and error what was helpful to eat and what to stay away from to minimize my symptoms, and then I was disciplined in following my regimen.
- I kept a daily gratitude journal.

How others supported me
- My children had a rotation of calling, so that one of them called me every day.
- Two friends who were cancer survivors acted as my coaches, being my sounding boards and guiding my actions along the path to diagnosis and treatment.
- Two long-term friends served as points of contact to coordinate with people who wanted to help, kind of my personal traffic cops, which was super helpful.
- I experienced an amazing outpouring of love and support from my family and many other friends.
- Several friends came to sit with me during my chemo infusions, which helped calm my nerves and made me feel supported.
- My friends put together a fund to pay for massages; I had a massage therapist come to my house to give me massages so it would be more sterile, and I was able to get a massage every week during treatment.
- After all of my procedures and treatments, a friend bound all of the CaringBridge messages into a book.

Helpful tips
- If you know someone experiencing a cancer diagnosis, offer to go with them to appointments to take notes if it feels appropriate; the trauma of hearing a cancer diagnosis limited my ability to comprehend, and I didn't feel like my brain was

processing at a normal level, so having notes enabled me to review the details later.

- If you want to be helpful and send articles, be sure to read anything before you send it, consider your intentions and whether it will be helpful or might be taken out of context; someone sent me a nutrition article about eating kale, and while I imagine the thought was intended to be positive, I took it to mean I had caused the cancer by eating the wrong food.
- Reach out and say hello when someone you know has been diagnosed or is going through treatment; touch base from time to time, as saying nothing is hurtful to cancer patients.
- If you have not experienced a cancer diagnosis, don't say you understand what your friend is going through; while well intended, it comes across as inauthentic.
- Learn how to advocate for yourself every single day and learn how to trust that you know what you need.
- When you go to a hospital or outpatient facility, be conscious of where you park; know that the parking for radiation or infusion is important, as sometimes patients don't have the energy to walk more than a few steps.

Surprising experiences

Think about the comments you make when you see someone who you think has cancer and try to be considerate of how they will be received. Two such experiences were deflating and devastating, at a time when I was just gaining strength and feeling good about my chances of survival. I was in the bathroom, about to shower at the YMCA one day after my workout. I took off my wig, something I had just become comfortable wearing. A woman next me said, "Oh do you have breast cancer? My friend died of breast cancer." Just as I was gaining belief that I would survive, hearing those words devastated me. Another example was from one night when I was attending a work event, as I socialized with clients and business colleagues. I was talking to one woman, who had not heard I had cancer. I had just finished explaining my story and where I was when she said, "Aren't you scared all the time? Oh, my goodness, how could you not have a bilateral mastectomy? You are going to die." I looked at her and walked away, as her words permeated my being. My upbeat mood plummeted to despair, wondering if she could be right.

The most uplifting experience that surprised me was the support from my community. My family, friends, and coworkers amazed me with their ongoing kindness. I felt like I had an army of people propping me up every day, which gave me such strength.

RONN'S STORY

———•——●——•———

It was early August of 2014, and I had not been feeling like myself for a few weeks—my stomach felt full and bloated, and I was experiencing sharp pains shooting through my stomach every day or two. My appetite had diminished, and I had lost my desire for food. I was sleeping in an elevated state in our bed to keep the acid reflux in check. At the same time, my wife and I were busy preparing for our four children—ages seven, eight, fourteen, and fifteen—to go back to school, buying supplies, and making sure summer homework was complete. My focus was on my family and work, and I kept putting off my health. A few weeks later, I noticed that my symptoms were still there—my stomach still felt full of fluid, and my desire for food had not returned. I really enjoy food and knew this was a signal of something serious. I mentioned it to my wife, and she added that she had noticed me looking a little yellow at times.

I decided to walk over to my neighbor's house. He is an emergency room physician who also worked at the urgent care center. He recommended I come see him the next day. When I arrived for the appointment, the nurse took my vital signs. My friend examined me and then recommended some blood work. The nurse drew blood, and I was to come back the next day for results. When

I returned the following day, he pulled up the test results and explained everything to me. He said, "Ronn, I want to be able to help you here, but you have reached the limit of what we can take care of. You have two elevated numbers that warrant more investigation. I would recommend going to see your primary care doctor. You can take these results with you." He handed me the results, and I thanked him and went out to get in my car. My urgency to get answers was growing as my symptoms continued to intensify. Since I worked in healthcare, I understood how the system worked and had developed a close relationship with my physician and his office staff. I had their mobile numbers and their direct line, kind of like a bat phone. I dialed my physician's number and reached his nurse. I explained my symptoms and the results of my blood tests. The nurse was able to get the physician on the phone and he said, "So, Ronn, it's probably nothing to worry about, just a fluctuation in your lab values, maybe caused by stress. You're still working on that big deal to sell your company, right? So, here is what I want you to do. Go to CVS and buy the colonoscopy prep, it's a powder that you mix and drink. It really cleans out your system and will make the feeling of being bloated go away. Then call me afterward." I drove out of the parking lot and followed his orders.

I completed drinking the colonoscopy prep that night and by the next morning, I not only did not feel better, but I had woken up to a sense of my body being full of fluid, I was belching more than ever and was now nauseous. I decided to go see my primary care physician. It was the first day of school, and my wife was a teacher's assistant in the elementary school, so I went to the appointment alone. My doctor was perplexed by my symptoms and how they had intensified instead of decreasing. He was aware of my family history of gallbladder issues with my father, so he ordered an ultrasound of my gallbladder. The nurse came in and recommended I go downstairs to the radiology office, where she had faxed the order. I was pretty distracted by how I felt so I didn't pay much attention as I rode the elevator down to the second floor. As I walked into the office, I observed that the waiting room was full of people, and every chair was occupied, something I had never experienced before at this office. I went up to the desk and learned that the computers were not working. I asked the woman at the front desk, "What radiology office has the shortest waiting line right now?"

She gave me a puzzled look and probably wondered how I had known what to ask for. She said, "I can set you up in an hour at the office in Brentwood. It's about a twenty-minute drive from here." I thanked her for working with me and asked her to forward the orders to the other location.

As I drove to Brentwood, I talked to my business partner on the phone and worked through some issues related to the upcoming sale of our company. I arrived at the office, thinking that what was causing my symptoms was my gallbladder. After all, my father had experienced gallbladder issues and had just had his removed. I mostly wanted to figure out what was wrong so I would start feeling better. My wife and daughters had been very patient with my edgy tone, and I wanted to get back to being myself. I walked into the office and checked in. As I sat in the waiting room, I caught up on work email on my phone and made a couple of calls. I texted my wife to let her know what was happening next. Time passed quickly as I focused on taking care of my business affairs. I was called back to the ultrasound room and lay down on the table. The technician started the ultrasound as I watched the screen. Everything seemed normal until she stopped the procedure and asked to be pardoned while she ran next door "for a sec." I thought nothing of it.

When she returned, she wasn't alone. She had gone to the cardiology office and brought back a doctor who introduced himself and began to give me unexpected news. He said, "Ronn, it looks like your pericardium is enlarged. That is the membrane enclosing your heart. I want to impress upon you how serious this is. I don't really know how you are functioning today with this much fluid on your heart. I have called ahead to the hospital, and they are ready for you. It's important for you to go straight to the emergency room, tell them your name, and then go straight back to the cardiac cath lab. Don't wait." He handed me some papers as his words started to sink in. I felt numb and was still sorting out what I had just heard, although I knew it was important to follow his orders. *What could be causing my heart to swell up so much?* I wondered. His words kept repeating in my head as I walked to my car. I was on a mission to get to the hospital quickly, although I am not sure I should have driven in my condition. I called my wife to share the news and asked her to meet me at the hospital. We both were still in shock over what I had just learned. As I drove to the hospital, I called and left a message for my friend who happened to be the hospital's CEO. I asked him to "put in a good word" for his friend with the team in the cath lab. I was on autopilot as I pulled into the complex, not thinking of parking in front of the emergency room. I put my car in the parking deck as if it was a regular day and walked over to the emergency room.

I checked in at the front desk and gave my name. The man behind the desk stopped what he was doing and looked up at me. "Oh, so you are Ronn? Okay, come with me. I'll take you back to where you need to go." As I followed him, I was feeling grateful to have connections in the hospital and comforted that I would be well cared for. *How could this all be happening so quickly?* I wondered. I called my wife to tell her where we were.

I was led into the cath lab where I put on a gown and lay down. The nurse started an IV, and the anesthesiologist asked me several questions. The cardiologist came in and explained the procedure, saying he was going to drain the fluid. He said it would be important to see clear fluid once it was drained. I remember seeing a fuzzy picture of my wife walking in the room as the anesthesia dispersed through my veins and I went under. I learned later that the surgeon had drained a liter and a half of fluid off my heart, which helped relieve the pressure. He had also told my wife that he thought I had lymphoma, but he didn't want to tell me at this time as he wasn't sure. As my eyes opened, still groggy from the anesthesia, I could see the sack of fluid near my bed. I looked up and said to my wife, "Well that's not good. Isn't the fluid supposed to be clear?" She smiled without answering, and I dozed off again. The next time I opened my eyes, I could see the hospital walls passing by quickly as I was being wheeled down the hall with several nurses around me. I looked up and saw the sign—Intensive Care Unit (ICU). *Wow, something serious is going on, I am being moved to the ICU,* I thought.

During the four days I spent in the ICU, I constantly had a team of nurses and doctors around me, reading the monitors I was hooked up to and writing things down, coming and going. I looked up and gave my wife a puzzled look. She was at my side, holding my hand, and said, "Honey, you've been admitted to the ICU where they are going to stabilize your heart. For some reason, your body keeps producing fluid that is filling up the pericardium sack. They are trying to figure out how to stop it. I know this has all happened so fast. Know that I am not leaving your side. I love you." She took a deep breath and added, "Oh, and the kids are taken care of. They know you are here and that we're trying to figure out what's wrong. We have lots of people helping us, so no need to worry about anything." The ICU team continued to run tests on me for what felt like an eternity. I had a drainage line inserted into my chest, a PICC line in my neck, and an IV pump beeping in the background. I was then wheeled down quickly to the operating room for another surgical procedure with full anesthesia to install a thicker tube between my ribs.

Once I was stabilized, I was moved to a regular hospital room on the cardiology floor. After a couple of days, my body was still producing fluid, and the team had not figured out how to stop it. Since it was critical for my heart function not to have fluid in the pericardium, I was wheeled down to the operating room again. The surgeon cut a square in the pericardium called a "pericardial window," so if more fluid was produced, it would just drain into my abdominal cavity, and my body would naturally remove the fluid from there. It would not be able to build up again around my heart. I was starting to feel a little like I was on my bike riding back and forth to the operating room. On day four, I went again, this time for a procedure using an endoscope for viewing inside my esophagus, stomach, and small intestine, as the doctors were trying to figure out why I had been feeling bloated. The images showed several duodenal ulcers, all benign, nothing to be concerned about. The ulcers had been the cause of my stomach discomfort and loss of appetite. The doctor gave me some medicine that dissolved the ulcers in a short period of time. As I sat there thinking about the ulcers, I said a prayer of thanks. I know, it probably sounds strange to be thankful for ulcers, although in my case, the symptoms had led to the discovery of the fluid on my heart.

When I was back in my room, a new doctor came in and introduced himself as an oncologist with news to share. As my wife held my hand, he said, "Ronn, we found cancer cells in the fluid we drained. You have what's called adenocarcinoma of the lung. Because of the cancer cells in the fluid, your condition is pretty serious. It is considered stage IV. I'm happy to treat you here if you want, but one of the three best physicians in the world for your particular kind of cancer is here in Nashville. I can refer you." I lay there taking in his words. *He had said the word* cancer. *Wow. This is very serious,* I thought. *It's going to be a pain to deal with. And here I thought not feeling well was kind of normal, just part of getting older.*

Agitation started to fill my mind as I processed the events of the last two weeks, all having happened at such an accelerated pace. I looked up at the oncologist and said, "Wow, that's a lot to swallow. I'm still trying to get my head around the words you just said, although I know we need to act quickly. I am interested in seeing the oncologist you recommend. Thanks for referring me." After the doctor left, my wife and I hugged each other around the tubing as tears poured down our cheeks. Our life as we knew it had just changed direction forever. We decided to tell our two oldest daughters when they came over to the hospital later that night.

When the girls arrived, I said we had learned something about what was wrong and wanted to share it with them. I met with them one at a time, and each conversation sounded the same. "I have some tough news to share. Daddy has cancer. It's called adenocarcinoma of the lung, and it is stage IV."

My daughter asked, "Um, how many stages are there?"

I looked at her and said, "Four. While it sounds scary, it doesn't mean the worst. I'm going to get through this. We've got a good battle ahead of us." I still had several tubes around my chest, but I hugged each of them the best I could. Then they came over and sat on either side of the bed as we all held hands. A sobering feeling filled the air in my room as we looked at each other, taking in our new reality and what it might mean. Seeing the look of fear on their faces brought it all square into reality for me. I had cancer.

Two days later, I was discharged with an oxygen tank and a cannula, which is a thin tube that goes around your nose, as I needed supplemental oxygen to keep my levels in normal range. My wife and I knew it was time to tell our two younger children, a boy and a girl. We sat them down after school and I said, "Daddy is sick. I will need to go through some treatment. We are going to get through this. I don't want you to worry." They each looked at each other and back at me. As they sat there, I could almost see their minds thinking through what sick meant. Sick to them at this point meant I would get well. I could tell by the look on their faces that they thought everything was going to be okay. I hugged both of them and said I loved them.

The mood in the house turned somewhat somber, and the days of wrestling on the sofa were gone for now. It was tough for my children to see their strong dad walking around the house with tubes and machines. I moved through my days in a bit of a fog, still questioning my new reality, until my business partner showed up and shifted my focus. Work gave me something to distract me, to take my mind off my diagnosis. He came to the house every day to work with me on the business deal. Our company was still in the nascent stages of forming, pre-client and pre-revenue. We had a larger company interested in investing in our concept and had several details to work through together.

I was able to get an appointment with the oncologist within a few days of leaving the hospital because of the seriousness of my condition and having a personal referral. Knowing that we needed to act fast, the office also scheduled an appointment at the hospital to have a port-a-cath inserted into my vein. A port-a-cath is used to draw blood and administer drugs, a typical next step in the treatment process. My procedure was on the same day as my appointment with the oncologist. I remember waking up in recovery, groggy from the anesthesia after the procedure, and looking at my watch. *Oh no, it took longer than I thought. I have to go now,* I realized.

I convinced the nurse to let me leave early so I could make my appointment, and my wife drove us over to the office. My sister and brother joined us there. A strikingly young gentleman came into the exam room and introduced himself. After discussing how I ended up in his office, he looked at me and said, "Well, Ronn, you have cancer. It is stage IV, adenocarcinoma of the lung." I swallowed, making a loud gulping sound, as if I was hearing this for the first time. I felt bewildered hearing this news again, not from a point of feeling defeated, but from the perspective of knowing there would be a tough road ahead. The doctor explained what would happen next—more scans and reviews by other specialists he trusted—before he could develop a definitive treatment plan. It took several weeks before we had a final plan.

One of the memorable moments from this time period was having lunch with my friend, a cancer survivor from 1985. Only a few days after I was discharged from the hospital, he called me and declared, "I'll be over to pick you up in thirty minutes for lunch; get dressed." That statement sounded more like a directive than an invitation, so I got dressed. During our time together, he gave me some valuable insight into what to expect during treatment, which I referred back to often. He looked at me and said, "People you know are going to show themselves in different ways to you as you walk this path. I experienced two subsets, whether they were my friends and family or just acquaintances. One subset is going to show up for you, regardless of the time of day or the condition you are in, and give their undying love and support, whatever you need. The second subset may be people who love you dearly, but they will not be to handle Ronn with cancer. They don't know how to cope with your being sick or their own fears of what might happen to them. They don't want to see it in you and will pull back into the shadows and withdraw. It doesn't mean they love you less. It is more about them than you." As I walked my path with cancer, I did indeed experience these two camps. Knowing ahead of time enabled me to weather the surprises during my treatment. He had sage advice that helped me to understand more about people's reactions as I endured cancer treatment.

The hardest part for me was watching my children come to terms with Daddy being sick. As a parent, I wanted to shield my children from experiencing harm or hurt, and here I was, helpless in my ability to change the situation. The cancer diagnosis was real and far reaching in its impact on my family. I had lost a lot of weight in a short period of time, and the tubes and machines were a constant reminder of my illness. My two older daughters had been Google searching about my diagnosis and had read some hard things about my chances of survival and what I might be like during treatment. One daughter became withdrawn and the other daughter had almost daily emotional outbursts over things like finding the milk jug empty in the refrigerator. Every day was an emotional rollercoaster once they came home from school. Then they started to question me, thinking they weren't getting the full story of what was happening. They even asked to go to an appointment with me. When I took them one day, they asked to meet with the doctor without me, which I allowed. We were operating in foreign territory here, and there were no ground rules. They asked the doctor how long I had to live. He said he didn't know, although he thought it would be a long time. The discussion seemed to help calm their fears to some degree.

Treatment Experience

When the scans and reviews were complete, my oncologist was ready to share the treatment plan. I learned I wasn't a candidate for surgery or radiation at that time. He wanted to shrink the seven tumors in the middle of my chest. He decided on Carboplatin as my chemotherapy drug regimen, in conjunction with Alimta. I started chemotherapy treatment in early September of 2014 and was scheduled to have an infusion every three weeks for seventy-eight weeks. I affectionately called the drug regimen "battery acid," as it felt like it was totally cleaning out my system. Every time I went in for an infusion, I would end up in bed for two to three days. I mostly felt extreme fatigue and weakness, and sometimes had a hard time catching my breath. I would regain strength and feel better during weeks two and three, before having another infusion. My wife was a devoted partner through it all, going with me to every appointment and every infusion, which gave me strength and comforted me. One of the positive side effects of the chemotherapy I was on was it completely cleared up the psoriasis I had. Psoriasis is an autoimmune disease that I had been diagnosed with many years before.

Early on in my treatment, I questioned why this was happening to me and questioned my decisions, although I didn't allow myself to stay in that space for long. I instinctively knew I needed to shift my focus to surviving the cancer. I decided a mantra would be helpful to remind me to turn my attitude around. I landed on, "Rally, rally, rally!" I even thought about getting it tattooed on my forearm so I could see it as an immediate reminder. (I didn't get the tattoo.) I had hit rock bottom, but I was going to feel better in an hour and even better the next day. I kept a positive outlook from that day forward, using my new mantra to motivate me, although I kept it to myself in the beginning.

With the full days of raising four children while we both worked, time to invest in my relationship with my wife was limited. We didn't make it a priority until I was diagnosed with cancer. When I was feeling stronger in October, we took a trip to the Florida Panhandle, just the two of us, for a long weekend. We held each other a lot, had deep conversations about what it all meant, and cried every day, as we felt and processed the emotion of the past few months and how much our lives had changed. We took walks on the beach and watched sunsets, comparing each one to the next. We talked about how we had a big fight ahead of us and agreed to tackle it side by side, as partners, and hold our family first above all else. I shared with her how I had been questioning why this was happening to me and how I had come up with, "Rally, rally, rally!" to motivate me. She was delighted I had shifted to focusing on the positive, believing I would survive. We also talked about how grateful we each felt that I was still here and how God had protected me through the process of uncovering the cancer. We reflected on how amazed we were with the undying support and love of our family and friends. And we started a new tradition, something new for us, taking selfies spontaneously and to mark certain events. A picture speaks a thousand words, and these selfies are some of my greatest treasures of my treatment experience.

By Thanksgiving, the scans showed only four tumors, and the ones remaining were shrinking in size. The doctor continued the Carboplatin and Alimta treatment regimen as I still had two more rounds. In January 2015, he stopped the Carboplatin and kept the Alimta, keeping me on that regimen for a total of eighteen months. With each scan every three months, my results kept getting better. Some of the tumors had disappeared and the others were either stable or shrinking. My body had adjusted enough that I would go in for the Alimta infusion and then be able to go to work; my symptoms had become mild and manageable.

In August of 2016, my condition had improved beyond my doctor's expectations. He finally said, "Here's the deal: I am going to have a conversation I have never had before. If you were to present today with your cancer, I would suggest you do radiation in addition to chemotherapy. There have been recent studies that show this helps." My doctor was determined to throw all his tools at my cancer, trying to make the last two tumors in my lymph nodes go away. He said, "We've got it down to almost nothing. We're going to put our foot on the throat of this cancer and knock it out."

While I continued with the Alimta infusions every three weeks, my doctor decided to add the Carboplatin back into the regimen along with IMRT radiation. I went a week before radiation started so they could build a cradle specifically for my body to hold me in the same position every time, trying to take the movement variable out of the equation. My treatments were every day, five days a week for six weeks. When I started radiation, I quickly noticed the same people in the room as I showed up at same time every day. We laughed and called it our country club, and the guys I was with were my foursome, all older guys who had prostate cancer. "Mr. Three Forty" was my nickname given by the technician, as that was my radiation time.

One guy was especially memorable. I would work hard to get him talking about something other than being sick or the treatment we were going through. When I did, he would shine brightly from the inside. It was during radiation that I met Greg and Kristi, whose story is also featured in this book. It felt like a divine appointment as I learned about his story. A budding friendship ensued, and I was able to be a sounding board for Greg as he dealt with his new diagnosis.

Through my conversations during radiation, I saw two different types of patients emerge. One saw the treatment as a step in the process, something he or she was going through on the path to beat the cancer or do everything trying. The other had more of a victim mentality, a sense that this was going to defeat them. I was part of the first group, always believing I would survive. Right from the start, the radiation impact was major. It burned my esophagus and made it hard to eat or drink. I forced myself to drink Ensure every morning and night. That was only eight hundred calories total so, as you might imagine, I lost a lot of weight during that time. I was grateful to finish the radiation treatments in September of 2016 and continued to get the Carboplatin and Alimta chemotherapy infusions every three weeks for eighteen weeks, and then just Alimta every three weeks for another eighteen months.

In December of 2017, I had one hot spot in my upper chest. My doctor recommended a focused radiation treatment, called SBRT. Even though it was in a difficult place, the radiologist would be able to "sharp shoot" it and take care of it. It was a highly targeted approach, focused on a square centimeter, every day for five days. I had to wear a vest that would immobilize my arms against my sides so I couldn't move. They placed four little mirrors on my chest—I could see the beam moving when I breathed. It was a surreal experience to go through, and I was grateful it only lasted a week. The following week, my business partner and I traveled to Denver to meet a client, and then went up to Keystone to ski over the weekend. I was skiing down the mountain and decided I wanted to share the experience with my doctor, show him how far I had come in three years. I pulled out my phone, put my poles under one arm, and pointed the camera down at my skis. Then I turned the camera back to my face and said, "How many of your patients do this?" Even though I had experienced a recurrence of the spot on my chest, I felt strong and was determined I would survive.

My doctor was at a panel with colleagues in December, and when I returned from my trip, he changed my treatment plan to add immunotherapy. Advances had been made in its use. When it first came out, immunotherapy was thought to work only for people with earlier stages of cancer. At the panel, my doctor learned that they were opening up the trial to stage III patients. Even though I was stage IV, he considered me a good candidate because I was doing so well. "We want to get you cancer free," he said. "Maybe we don't think of immunotherapy as a plan B like we did earlier on in your treatment." In January of 2018, I started on immunotherapy and stopped getting Alimta infusions. I continued to have scans every three months and still go back every three months at the writing of this book, which is why I glow in the dark today when you turn the lights off. My psoriasis started coming back over the course of six months. It became annoying, so my doctor decided to stop the immunotherapy.

Throughout my many years of treatment, I talked to new patients in the waiting room. I would try to share my story, encourage other people, and give them hope. Even if I was having a bad day, I believed it was important to be encouraging to others. It was equally important to me not to look like the face of cancer. Since my treatment period, I have looked out for people feeling the weight of cancer and helped out friends of friends. When I see them, I engage them and offer support. I learned early on through this process that if I am open to being useful along the journey, I could share my big heart with others and maybe lessen their pain. And that perspective led me to share my story with you.

I am confident that the power of prayer is why I am still living today. My grandmother died one month before turning 103 years old. She lived a full life up until her death. At her memorial service at the funeral home in Birmingham, Alabama, I met her pastor. I went up and introduced myself to him, saying "Hi, I'm Ronn Hollis."

His face lit up, and he said, "Oh, oh, I know of you, Ronn! I have been praying for you every day. I am part of this online pastoral group across five continents that shares stories and prays every day. Actually, people on five continents pray for you every day." I smiled and thanked him. In the midst of a sad circumstance, what he shared felt like a glimmer of light. I walked away, found a quiet place, and broke out sobbing, overcome with emotion by what I had just heard, proving the power of prayer.

I had moments over the past several years of wondering what if this or that happens next, but not hours. I never thought the cancer would take me away. When I went in last at the end of June 2019, my doctor was giddy. He smiled and said, "Do you realize it has been a year since you have been off all treatment?" I hadn't even thought about it.

Advice for Others

How I supported myself

- I focused every day on trying to be mentally tough and keep a positive outlook.
- Even if I had to force it, I would find a way to cry twice a day, in order to not swallow the emotion—I embraced it or created it if needed, by watching YouTube videos of soldiers surprising their children.
- I laughed a deep belly laugh twice a day, every day, by watching funny videos on YouTube, such as goofy animal tricks and comedians.
- I invested in what's important: My wife and I took regular trips to the beach, just the two of us.

How others support me

- Countless friends and family members supported me and my family through my years of treatment.
- Someone came and got my wife's car to get brakes replaced, paid for it, and brought it back.
- Someone showed up at the house and said here is our tithe—we are supposed to give it to you.
- The church started a meal train for our family—we didn't make a meal for three and a half months.
- A good friend came to mow our lawn for three years and never accepted any money.

Helpful tips

- If you know someone experiencing a cancer diagnosis, keep a positive attitude as you engage with them.
- Embrace emotions—it's okay to be vulnerable.
- Help others by talking through their diagnosis.
- Help a friend or family member create their own. "Rally, rally, rally!" to tell their body that it's time to get better now.

Surprising experiences

I would see people I knew, and when they heard I was still in treatment, they would say "When's it going to be over? I thought you were already done," or "Oh, are you still dealing with this? You've been doing this a long time." I would graciously reply, "Yes, I'm still in treatment. I have cancer, not the flu."

In March of 2018, I was having breakfast at a restaurant with some friends. A young woman, about thirty years old was having breakfast with her kids at a table near us. All of a sudden, she stood up, walked over to me, and said she needed to talk to me because God had asked her to share a message with me. She said, "I don't know if you have a faith or not. God just told me to tell you that he is going to attack your intellect. It is very specific for you, from God." Then she walked away. I still don't know what that message meant.

JENNIFER'S STORY

———•━●━•———

It was the end of March 2014, and I was sitting in my doctor's office for my annual checkup. As we were talking, she looked at me and said, "You know, Jennifer, given your family history, I think it would be good for you to go ahead and have a mammogram. Then, I want you to have an MRI in six months. I know you are only thirty-nine years old, and we typically recommend one starting at age forty, but let's go ahead and start now." It seemed like a reasonable approach to me. She wrote the order and the imaging center called to schedule it. I didn't think anything was out of the ordinary and arrived alone on April 3rd for my appointment. It was my first mammogram ever, and I was surprised at how painful it was, with all the manipulating of my tissue the technician did to get all the angles needed. When the mammogram was complete, the nurse recommended that I participate in genetic counseling due to my family history and walked me to another room. She asked me questions and put information into a computer. It appeared to be all about numbers. When she was finished gathering my details, she looked at me and said, "Good news, you actually don't have a risk of getting breast cancer." *Okay, that gives me a little peace of mind given my history,* I thought and breathed a sigh of relief. The radiologist called me the next day with the results, saying it was a normal mammogram. My doctor followed up with me to confirm the test results a few days later and recommended an MRI in October. She said it would be a good proactive step in managing my health to take these steps, given that both my mother and grandmother had been diagnosed with breast cancer and that my father had experienced cancer three times.

As I entered the month of May, I noticed that I was feeling dizzy and nauseous more and more during the day. One day I felt so bad that I went to the emergency room, feeling listless and extremely tired. The nurse took some blood and came back to start an IV. The doctor came in and said, "Something is strange because your white blood cells are off-the-chart high. I'm not sure why that is, although we are not finding anything else. Let's get some fluids in you. It may just be a stomach bug." The fluids gave me a little energy, and I drove home after a while. As I regained some strength, my phone rang a few days later. It was my mom telling me that my dad had an infection in his leg and would be having surgery soon. I quickly shifted my focus to him and arranged to fly to New Jersey to be with him the day before the surgery. My dad and I were very close. I was his only girl and the youngest child in the family. His health had been deteriorating, seemingly quickly, over the last several years. His dementia was also becoming more noticeable when I talked to him on the phone.

I landed in New Jersey and went straight to see him. When I walked into his room, I was shocked by the words that came out of his mouth. He looked at me and said, "Hi, I'm John." I took a step back and looked around me, wondering if there was someone else who had walked in behind me. I looked back at him and then realized how far his dementia had progressed. I held his hand and said, "Dad, I'm your daughter. You are the best father I could ask for. I love you so much." The next morning, I walked by his side as they wheeled him to the operating room. I was holding his hand and looking at him when I heard him say, in a hushed voice, "Thank you for being my daughter. I will always love you." A peace warmed my heart as his words permeated my mind. It was such a welcome change from the day before. I had to fly home after his surgery, while he was still in a medically induced coma, although he did regain consciousness a few days later. His health deteriorated significantly over the next two months, and on August 1, he died of heart failure. It turns out that I was the last person he talked to, and the loving words he shared with me were the last real words out of his mouth.

After he died, I struggled with the feeling that I had a deep hole in my heart. I cherished the last words he said and replayed them in my mind when I was feeling especially blue. I was still feeling tired and nauseous much of the time, although life with two children under the age of five, combined with running the household much of the time while my husband traveled for work, kept me distracted and busy. Before I knew it, October had arrived, and it was time to schedule the breast MRI that my doctor had recommended in April. I kept prioritizing other things in my life, and days floated by. I remembered I needed an MRI in November and was able to schedule it for the next day. I had the MRI on November 11, and the imaging center said they would call me back within forty-eight hours with the results. Two days came and went. One of my friends knew that I'd had the MRI and when I saw her at school every day, she would ask me if I had the test results yet. This went on for about two weeks. If my dear friend hadn't followed up, my situation would have had a different outcome. I am eternally grateful for her persistence. Our budding friendship started with the cancer and grew into a long-lasting beautiful friendship through this experience. A few days later, I was taking a shower one night and doing my breast self-exam. As I washed under my left arm, my fingers ran across a lump. *Ouch.* I jumped a little as it hurt so badly to touch it. The lump was about the size of a golf ball. *Hmm, that wasn't there yesterday. I am surprised it hurts so badly. It must be an ingrown hair. I will call the doctor tomorrow to make sure*, I thought. I fell into bed and went to sleep quickly, exhausted from the day.

The next morning, I picked up my phone and called my doctor's office, reaching her nurse. She pulled up my chart and there was silence on the other end of the phone for what felt like hours. Then she said, "Jennifer, I just looked at your MRI results, and there is something showing in your left breast. I'm sorry no one called you. Let's get you over to the imaging center today for an ultrasound."

My heart was racing as I heard these words. "What did you just say?" I asked. "I want to make sure I understand."

The nurse replied, "There is a spot on your MRI. I am very sorry again about the mix-up." All of a sudden, I became numb as I checked my calendar. She said she would call me back with a time for the ultrasound in a few minutes. I was desperate to move quickly and get some answers. I called my neighbor two doors down, although I didn't know her or her story. "Hi," I said. "I live two houses down and need help. I need to go to the doctor for some tests; would you be able to watch my son for a little bit?" She graciously offered to help and came down five minutes later.

I had just moved to Denver, Colorado, from New Jersey the year before and didn't know that many people, so I went alone. As I drove to the imaging center, my heart was beating twice as fast as normal. I kept wondering why no one had called as anger filled my thoughts. And here I had thought no news was good news—boy was I wrong. I arrived at the center, checked in, and the nurse called me right back. She said I would have a diagnostic mammogram and then an ultrasound on my left side. *What, a mammogram also? I was only supposed to have an ultrasound. Okay, this is sounding a little serious and here I am by myself.* Chills permeated my spine as I walked towards the mammogram machine. The technician moved through the tests fairly quickly. Everything was moving at such a fast pace I barely had time to think about the transitions. Then I was called back to talk to the radiologist. I walked into the room and saw the doctor sitting there, looking at the screen. He introduced himself, and then started to explain what he was seeing on the screen. He said he had found three lumps on my chest on the left side, and they were most likely cancerous. I blurted out, "What do you mean three lumps? I only found one."

He looked at me with compassion and said, "Yes, I do see three lumps. Two are on your chest. I would recommend a biopsy to learn more."

I gulped as the words settled into my brain. *A biopsy, okay, that means something might be wrong. That's a lot more than an ingrown hair.* He told me that the nurse was scheduling the biopsy, and she would be in soon with the details. He left the room. I was still a little bewildered with the words "you need to have a biopsy." I took a deep breath. *Was this really happening?* The nurse came in and said my biopsy was scheduled for December 5.

I drove back to my house in a daze and walked to my neighbor's house. When she opened the door, she looked at me and said, "Are you okay?" I broke down and started crying uncontrollably right there in the entrance to her house. She wrapped her arms around me and said softly, "You are going to get through this." After I calmed down, she invited me in and shared her story. She was a breast cancer survivor and had experienced a double mastectomy. She recommended her oncologist and surgeon highly, which I appreciated. I met her daughter, who offered to help if needed. While our relationship was in the nascent stages of forming, I felt covered in love and support.

My husband had recommended that we go away for Thanksgiving to the mountains and experience a change of scenery. We were able to leave early on Monday the week of Thanksgiving. I was so grateful for his thoughtfulness. Getting away to the mountains really helped cleanse my soul.

On December 5, I went to back to the clinic for the biopsy by myself. I was feeling disconnected from my body and was nervous about what would happen next. The radiologist prepped the area and then started the procedure. I could feel a clipping sensation inside my left breast and said, "Hey, I can feel this!" He continued with the second one and I grabbed his arm and shouted, "Holy Mother of God, I feel you snipping in there. Stop! You need to numb my whole breast now!" He listened to me this time and stopped to numb my whole breast. Then he continued, cutting samples of the tissue from the last tumor. My stomach was in knots as I watched the screen and looked back at him. It felt as if time was suspended as I focused intently on what he was doing, lost in the moment. Then I heard him say my name. He was finished with the procedure. He said he would send the tissue to the lab and would call in a couple of days with the test results.

Here it was Friday, so I would be waiting until at least Monday. I kept replaying the feeling of the clipping in my mind as I drove home. I felt dizzy, and my left arm was starting to ache. When I got home, I found my husband home early from work. I told him about the biopsy, and that we would hear something in a few days. He asked me if I was okay, and I said yes, I just felt sore. He reminded me that we had his office Christmas party that night and needed to leave soon, something that had slipped my mind given the recent tests. I was grateful to have something else to focus on, a distraction from the events of the last few days.

At the party, I did my best to appear normal and strong as we talked to his coworkers, although the reality that I was waiting on biopsy results would pop up in a distant part of my mind when there was a lull in activity. That night, I fell asleep quickly, exhausted from the procedure and the mental gymnastics going on in my mid. My husband had to leave on Sunday for work, so it felt like a compressed weekend, overfull with activities and caring for our young children.

On Monday afternoon, I was in my room trying to rest when the phone rang. I can remember that moment like it was yesterday, the jeans I was wearing and the way I was lying on the bed in my room. It was 1:50 in the afternoon. My son was taking a nap, and my daughter was at school. I answered the phone and on the other end, the radiologist said, "Jennifer, I am calling to tell you the biopsy results. The tests came back malignant. You have cancer, although we don't know what kind yet." Almost immediately, I said, "Okay" and hung up, as a blood-curdling scream came out of my mouth. I started sobbing uncontrollably. My breath was short, and I began to hyperventilate, gasping for air. I started pacing the floor. *Oh no, this is the worst. I am going to die. Why God, why me? This isn't fair! What is happening? You know I just lost my father a few months before, and now this? Really?*

I dialed my husband's phone number to tell him, even though it was almost nine at night in London where he was. "Hi honey, the doctor's office called, and I have some bad news. I do have cancer." My sobbing continued as the words sunk in for us both.

He said, "Okay, it's going to be fine. Everything is going to be okay. I will come home as soon as possible. I love you." As I hung up, I could feel my face turn a bright red and get hot as I thought about God and why he let this happen, after all I had been through. I started to question my Catholic faith as the anger welled in my mind. After about ten minutes, something inside me shifted my focus, and I started to regain my composure. I took several deep belly breaths and thought, *This is stopping. No more tears. I am going to have a plan. I need to do something. Call someone. Not just anyone, someone who can help.*

A calming feeling pulsed through my veins as I dialed the number for my mother's breast cancer surgeon in New York. Having lived in New Jersey all my life, my medical history was with doctors there, so it felt easiest to start my treatment back in the New York area. I also had a feeling I would be able to get in quicker as a result. Something was giving me strength and composure all of a sudden. I was surprised to hear the office was still open, as it was two hours later there. I was able to talk to the nurse, explain what had happened, and tell her I needed help.

She said, "Jennifer, we will definitely fit you in and, yes, we need to move quickly given your family history. If you can get to town, we could see you this Thursday. I'll put the front desk on the phone to work out the details. Hang in there." Taking action felt powerful and gave me hope. I needed a plan, and within minutes I had one. I shifted from being upset to scared to angry and then to confidence through action, all within fifteen minutes. I cried to the point where the tears would no longer come, to the point of exhaustion. My husband had called to tell me he would be back on Wednesday, which was the earliest he could fly home from London, and I let him know about my appointment. I called a couple of my close friends to share my test results and ask for their help with the kids. I needed to board a plane in two short days. As the plan started to take shape, hope started to come alive inside me. *I have a plan. I am going to act fast and beat this,* I thought as I started packing.

Comfortable that my children and the many details of their schedule were in capable hands, I flew alone to New Jersey on December 10. My mother met me at the airport, and we had a quiet night together at her house, talking about what I had just learned. She went with me to the office the next day, arriving thirty minutes early. I was anxious to learn more and understand what I was facing. As the doctor walked in the exam room and caught up with my mother, she looked at me and said, "Jennifer, we need to do more tests to know the type of breast cancer you have. From the biopsy results, I do know that this is a very aggressive type of cancer that is spreading rapidly, and we need to move fast." I sat there staring at her for what felt like thirty minutes. The words *very aggressive* kept spinning through my mind. She looked at me and said, "Given the situation, I would recommend surgery first. Let's talk about the kind of surgery and let me look at our schedule. And I would recommend having the genetic test for the BRCA gene. You can do that when you come back." I felt relieved and trusted this doctor, feeling more relaxed knowing what would happen next. The nurse came in and said they had an opening for the surgery on December 17, the following week. I was grateful to have it scheduled so soon and made plans to fly home on December 12.

The day before I flew to New Jersey for my surgery, my husband and I sat our daughter and son down to tell them what was going on. I looked at them and said, "Mommy is sick. I have cancer." My goal was to be transparent with them, every step of the way, even though they were young. My daughter was five years old and said, "What's that? Mommy, are you going to die?" I dug deep as I searched for an answer, knowing that my situation was not black-and-white, something a five-year-old believes at that stage in life. I replied, "I cannot promise that I won't die. I can say that I will fight every day to live for you. I don't know what is going to happen next." My daughter and son both came over and wrapped their little arms around me as tears rolled down our cheeks. That night after I put them to bed, I sat down and wrote each of them a letter, kind of a good-bye letter, I guess. I was leaving the next day and facing major surgery and wasn't sure of what would happen next. I am a planner and wanted to leave something behind, in the event that I didn't survive. I put both letters in the safe and told my husband to give one to each child on their eighteenth birthday.

As I waited for the details of my treatment plan to take shape, I thought back over the events of the past month. I had delayed having an MRI that my doctor had recommended, and why? Because keeping up with life and everyone else was more important than taking care of my health? As I processed all the steps that led me to my cancer diagnosis, I decided that my health was highly important, although I had not really prioritized focusing on myself before this point. I was always focused on other's needs. I also reflected on my blind faith that, since I had not heard back about my MRI results, everything was fine. An important lesson I learned is no news does not mean good news. I also learned the hard way how important it is to be your own advocate, to follow up on test results when you haven't heard.

Treatment Experience

I flew back to New York early in the morning of December 16 so I could complete all my pre-surgery tests and participate in genetic testing. Again, my mother picked me up and was with me as I prepared for surgery. The nurse at the hospital drew blood after my MRI, and then showed me where to go for the genetic testing. I walked in the office and met with a genetic counselor, who explained the three different levels of genetic tests and what each represented. I decided on one, and she told me what would happen next, and that it would take four weeks to get the results. The nurse came in the office and drew some blood. The genetic counselor explained that she would call when she had the results.

The next day, on the morning of December 17, I checked in early for surgery at the hospital. I had decided on a double mastectomy as I wanted to be proactive with my right side, given my family history. The minute I lay on the table, I started shaking with fear. The nurses were busy preparing me for the surgery and starting my medicine. My doctor noticed the look on my face and that I was shaking. She came over and put her hand on my arm, reassuring me that I would be fine and to close my eyes. The second I closed my eyes, I saw my dad's face, as clear as if he was in front of me, which calmed my nerves and gave me deep comfort and peace—my fears dissipated immediately. That is the last thing I remember. While I was under anesthesia on the operating table, the surgeon took tissue samples and put a rush on the lab results of my lymph nodes and the tumors. The breast cancer surgeon continued with the procedure and the plastic surgeon inserted what is called an "expander" in each breast to hold the muscles in place until my breast reconstructive surgery. While I was still on the table, my breast surgeon learned of the test results. The cancer had spread to some of my lymph nodes, so she removed nine on my left side and five on my right side. She also told me what kind of cancer I had—HER2 positive, and that it was stage III. When I woke up, I was covered from head to toe with hives and intense itching, and my skin was burning hot. I started scratching my skin so hard it was almost bleeding. The doctor quickly changed my pain medicine, and I learned I was allergic to morphine.

I stayed in the hospital for four days, and then went to stay with my mother to recover. The doctor wouldn't let me fly home yet. While it broke my heart to be away from my babies at Christmas, I was determined to act as fast as possible and give myself the highest chances of survival. My husband and I decided to celebrate Christmas when I got home, which was on New Year's Eve. Since our children were five and two, they didn't really notice. It was just another day for them, and while we celebrated, I was still weak and moved around the house slowly. As I moved into January of 2015, I started physical therapy every week for the lymphedema, a common side effect of having lymph nodes removed. The physical therapist recommended a sleeve to wear on my arm to keep the swelling down between visits. I would wear it when I worked out and when I flew on an airplane, and I still do. I also heard from the genetic counselor with the genetic test results in January. She said the test came back negative, that my cancer was not genetic. It was familial, just not genetic.

On Sunday before my first chemotherapy infusion, I decided to shave my head. I had shoulder length hair at the time. My goal was to be in control of what was left for me to control, and shaving my hair off before it fell out helped me feel in control. My children and husband and I gathered in my bathroom, and I put a sheet down on the floor under me. As I started shaving my hair, my daughter began singing the song from the movie *Frozen*, "Let it go." I felt so supported, which lightened the mood of why I was shaving my head. My children were watching my every move. When I offered to let them help, each of them would ask their dad, "Daddy is it okay? Are you sure?" After I finished shaving my head, my daughter and son were staring straight at me, looking at my head. Then my son said, "Can I touch your head? I want to feel your head." I reassured both of them that it was okay to touch my head. They both came over and rubbed my head.

Then my daughter said, "Is my hair going to fall out?" I told her not to worry about that.

To help them be prepared for what was to come, I said, "Mommy is going to get very sick, and I am not going to be the usual Mommy you know. I am going to have some really bad days." They hugged me and kept rubbing my head. I had shaved it down to a super short buzz cut. After two days of staring at me and rubbing my head, they both moved on. I imagine at their age the transition was over, and they accepted that Mommy was bald, no big deal.

I started chemotherapy infusions on February 9, and my doctor recommended I get the drug regimen called Red Devil. I would go in every other Thursday, and by Saturday, I would be deathly ill, nauseous and lethargic, barely able to make it to my bathroom. My daughter would come in my room and sing "Amazing Grace" to me every Saturday. At my second infusion, I asked my doctor if the rest of my hair was going to fall out. I think I even said, "I will choke you if I did this and my hair was not coming out." He said yes and sure enough, after my second infusion, the rest of my hair did start to fall out. I went to my gym to work out the following week and remembered there was a hair salon inside. I found the salon and walked in, finding a woman who was available standing by a chair. I caught her eye and said, "I am going through cancer treatment and would like you to finish shaving my hair off, will you do that?"

She looked at me and nodded, motioning for me to sit in her chair. As she picked up her razor, she said, "I had someone in my life who died of breast cancer. This cut will be my treat to you." She proceeded to shave the small amount of hair left on my head.

When we would be in the grocery store while I was going through treatment, my daughter would say to people who would walk by and look at us, "Don't look at my mother, she is sick with cancer." Those were sobering words to hear come out of my five-year-old's mouth. I was acutely aware of the looks on these people's faces as she spoke those words. Yes, I was a cancer patient and likely looked like one. It was such a humbling experience to see the way they looked at me and know this was my reality. Pretty soon all the rest of the hair on my arms and legs fell out. I had skin as soft as a newborn baby. It kind of felt like my body was regenerating from the inside out as a result of the chemo drugs.

Rounds three and four of chemotherapy were the toughest on my body. I was throwing up and couldn't keep anything down, not even water. My daughter would bring me her pink "throw-up" bucket. She was only five years old, yet she shifted into helping me almost instinctively. I gave her a big hug and thanked her for helping me feel better. She looked at me and said, "That's all right, Mommy. It's going to be okay. I was born to help you fight cancer." I felt those words down in the depths of my soul, amazed at her ability to speak so articulately at such a young age. While she was willing to help me, I could see concern on her face. This experience definitely matured her faster than most five-year-olds, although it also taught her compassion. Life was strained in our family with me being out of commission as a mom, especially as much as my husband traveled. I was grateful to have my neighbor's daughter who lived two doors down and was old enough to drive. She was willing to help, so I hired her to help care for my children, which was her primary responsibility, and then do chores around the house and drive me to my appointments as well. Being such a strong, independent woman made it really difficult to accept my neighbor's help. In the past, I had not let anyone help me. This young woman was a life saver to me and our family, and I am deeply grateful for her loving kindness and willingness to step in and take over when I could no longer manage.

I always had a special chemo bag prepared the night before my infusion appointment and was ready for battle the next day. In my bag I had a warm blanket, a twenty-four-ounce cup for ice water, my journal, and my music. I built friendships with a group of fellow cancer patients who had infusions at the same time on Thursday. Several of their stories are included in this book—Robyn, Nikki, and Kim. We named ourselves the "Chemo Warriors." We helped support each other and held the positive space together, focused on moving forward and healing. My heart would expand each time I saw my friends during infusions. We formed a special type of bond, all enduring the vulnerable experience that is chemotherapy. I would suck on ice pops while getting my infusions of the Red Devil drug. One side effect I had was sores in my mouth, throat, and esophagus. It was difficult to find anything to eat that didn't burn my mouth.

Through trial and error, I learned to swish plain Greek yogurt around in my mouth for a few minutes, and the live cultures helped kill the sores. I was not able to drink shakes because the sugar in them would burn my mouth, so the yogurt trick was a life saver. I learned to eat a half sandwich midway through the infusion, which lessened my nausea and helped increase my energy level. I would also go in the next day to get an IV flush of saline fluid. Chewing on sour gummy worms helped me manage the strong taste in my mouth from the saline, as the IV increased my energy levels tenfold. Every chemo infusion would take its toll on my body as it built up in my system. When my body had rallied to recover from the previous treatment, then it would be time for another infusion with more drugs. I learned that rubbing coconut oil on my scalp in the shower helped decrease the dry scalp and helped my hair grow back thick and quicker. Despite the side effects, with my warrior group's support and positive attitude, I shifted my focus to managing life one day at a time, one drug at a time, one breath at a time through the rest of my treatment.

Following chemotherapy, I endured thirty-five radiation treatments. I went in every weekday for seven weeks. Radiation was much easier on my body than the chemotherapy. As I was starting radiation, I was determined to be in control of what I could control, meaning preparing well and taking care of myself after the treatment to lessen the side effects. Through trial and error, I figured out that rubbing Aquaphor on my chest right after my treatment in the morning and then again in the afternoon was helpful and lessened the burning impact of the radiation. I used an Australian nut cream called Tamanu Oil at night as the treatments continued. My last seven sessions were the hardest to endure. They are called blast—the machine is literally lying right on top of your breast. I could feel it burning my insides to the bone. Beyond the intense burning during the procedure, the only radiation side effects I experienced were extreme fatigue and constant thirst. I increased my water intake threefold, on top of my extra water intake due to living at a high altitude.

As I was going through all my treatments, I had many friends offering to help me. My cancer experience led me to one of my best friends today. She had a son the same age, and she became another mother to my son during my treatment. She would send videos and pictures of the special moments I would miss. I am so grateful to her for our friendship and our forever bond. At the beginning of my cancer treatment, I thought I was Wonder Woman and that I would be able to handle everything, all by myself. When I finally let my guard down and started letting others help me, I felt lighter and healed more quickly. It truly takes a village to get through breast cancer, and it is important to be vulnerable and let others help. It gave me peace to know my friends were there when I needed them. Having all the love and support is what helped me get through each day of this battle with cancer. I still prefer to do a lot myself, although I am open to letting people help now. I developed deeper friendships that are longer lasting through being vulnerable and accepting help from others. The process also made me more accepting of others, knowing we each have a story and may be fighting our own battle silently.

What most people don't talk about is the side effects that show up one, two, three years down the road. At year three, I started having trouble with my circulation and still do today. I experienced dry eyes, insomnia, and neuropathy in my feet, and I lost my hearing in my right ear. I have also experienced bad BPPV vertigo from time to time. Since my doctor said there isn't a cure for this, he recommended the Epley maneuver, which helped. While I had experienced migraines in the past before my cancer diagnosis, I started having vestibular migraines in the past year, which have impacted my balance and are debilitating and painful. I went to a neurologist recently who prescribed Botox, which is helping tremendously. All of these side effects constantly remind me that I was a cancer patient who endured life-altering treatments.

While I grew up in the Catholic Church and went to a Catholic school, this experience definitely challenged my faith in a deep way. I transitioned from questioning God in the early stages to feeling completely grounded with a hope for a bright future. While I used to go to church some, I now go every week and light candles for my friends and loved ones. The church has an amazing candle room where I feel supported and loved. Praying daily helped to expand this feeling of comfort, which kept me going through the ups and downs. Through every step, every minute, every hour, I felt like my dad was with me, giving me strength to endure and persevere. Praying daily helped to expand this feeling of strength and comfort, which kept me going through the ups and downs.

After my first ten-minute pity party, I shifted to focusing on the positive, believing that I was not going to die from the cancer. And the minute I started thinking about being sad, I would change what I was focusing on and think positive. Something that helped me shift was going to the gym every day, even if for only for five or ten minutes. Getting up and moving would help me feel alive. I would also run on the treadmill sometimes and visualize the cancer leaving my body, like water melting from an ice cube. I had so much to live for; there was no other choice in my mind.

I experienced two types of loved ones on my journey. One type was the people who were there every step of the way. The second type was the people who did not show up at all, which felt hurtful and upset me. While I knew instinctively that it was their issue, it was still tough. I learned how important it was to ask for what I needed from my husband and not to assume he knew. Communication is critical, every step of the way.

The hardest part of this experience for me was when it was over—when I was done with all the activity. My first-year post treatment was the hardest, remembering every anniversary of the "firsts"—the first time I learned of my diagnosis or when I had my surgery. I was so afraid of every little symptom and wondered if I needed to have each one checked out. I was always looking over my shoulder and focusing on my numbers after every test. By the second year, I started living my life again, began experimenting, and was willing to try new things. I started planning for my future and focused forward on what exciting thing lay ahead for me and my family. Given my family history and the aggressive nature of my type of cancer, my doctor asked to follow me for twenty years. December 17, 2019 was my five-year mark from my surgery. Thankfully, the cancer experience no longer holds weight in my mind. My experience made me stronger than ever, and no fears can stand in my way. Now, my focus on positivity is what pushes me forward in life each day.

Advice for Others

How I supported myself
- I was determined to try things to lessen the side effects of all the treatments; as a result, I was able to manage most with minimal impact compared to other people.
- I did some kind of exercise every day, even if it was for five minutes; I would go to the gym or run on the treadmill.
- I would pray every day, for my healing, my family, and my friends.

How others supported me

- I had many friends come help with the children, make dinners for my family, clean my house, and take my children to activities and school and pick them up again.
- My sister-in-law gave us a very generous gift certificate for home-delivered meals that was one of the best gifts for us, as my husband was able to choose the food with minimal effort.

Helpful tips

- Food smells are challenging for many cancer patients—if you are cooking for one, keep the food very bland.
- Think about the comments you make when you see someone who you think has cancer and try to be considerate of how it will be received. Hearing these comments from people I knew and total strangers did not sit well with me and led me to question my positive outlook:
    - "Is this terminal, are you going to live?"
    - "Wow, you have so much drama in your life!"
- Pay attention when your animals act different around you; my German shepherd would sniff my mother's right armpit when she had cancer and used to sniff my left side, under my armpit near my chest, until I was diagnosed; he has not done it since.
- If you want to do something, set up a meal train and put in dietary restrictions
- Go buy household staples like toilet paper, paper towels, and laundry soap, all things people need, and then drop them off on the front porch.
- Wait until the person with the diagnosis reaches out to ask for advice; try not to offer advice or ask for them to call you, which feels like another job to the person with cancer.

Helpful tips for cancer patients

- Get a journal and keep track of all of your side effects between your appointments; it will help you be able to share details, as chemotherapy messes with your memory and continues for about a year.

- Bring someone with you when you go to doctor's appointment to take notes.
- For those going through radiation, rub Aquaphor on the radiation site right after and then in the afternoon, then tamanu oil at night; increase your water intake at least twofold.
- For chemotherapy infusions, bring a soft blanket, a journal, a big glass for ice water, and a snack to eat after the first drug; eat sour gummies to help get rid of the taste from flushing the port on the day after the infusion, as it tastes like dirty salt water.
- Put coconut oil on your eyes before bed if they are dry.
- Two books to read—*Chicken Soup for the Soul of Cancer Patients* and *Just Get Me Through This: A Practical Guide to Coping with Breast Cancer*.
- If you lose your hair, rub coconut oil on your scalp when in the shower; let it soak in.
- If you are a side sleeper, buy two oblong neck pillows to support your new body parts while you sleep, putting one in the middle of your back to help keep you on your side and the other in between your implants.
- It is also important to not make any major decisions until a year after chemotherapy treatment has ended; life starts to take shape again at that point, becomes clearer and normal again.

Surprising experiences

When I went in for my third chemotherapy infusion and was walking to my chair, it felt like the calm before the storm. I walked past another patient, and she turned and said, "You have lots of spirits around you, and they are all in the hallway out there."

I turned around and looked out in the hallway, then looked back at her inquisitively, as I didn't see anyone. "Thank you very much," I said and continued walking to my chair. I thought to myself, *Okay, lady, thank you very much. I don't know what is in your cocktail today, but I don't need any of that. I appreciate your spirits, have a nice day.*

When I walked past her, she grabbed my arm and said, "But there is one person, your father, who is here for you and is going to get you through this. He wanted me to tell you, 'Don't worry, my precious little girl, you going to get through this.' And he will be there for you." The words 'precious little girl' stopped me dead in my tracks. That is what my dad used to call me. There is no way this stranger could have known that or that my father had died, unless she was able to communicate with the other side. This experience gave me strength and validated my conviction that my dad's spirit was with me. I could trust myself and relax into the belief that all was well, and I would survive.

BILL K'S STORY

———— • ● • ————

I had just completed serving my twelfth legislative session as the senator representing the thirteenth district in Tennessee. I had settled into my normal summer routine of enjoying fishing at Center Hill Lake and running our family insurance business. I am an alumnus of Middle Tennessee State University (MTSU), and I had been asked to join an MTSU trip to China. We were preparing to leave at the end of July 2015. As I was packing, my tongue brushed over a bump inside my lower lip. *Ouch, that kind of hurt. I don't remember feeling that before,* I thought. I wondered if I needed to get it checked out before I left. I decided it would be a good idea since I was leaving the country. I called my doctor's office and left a message. When he called me back, he said, "Bill, it sounds like what you are describing is a clogged salivary gland. I would recommend stopping by Walgreens and buying some lemon drops. Sucking on the lemon drops will likely clear it up. Have a good trip." I thanked him and drove over to Walgreens. After eating the lemon drops on the plane, the bump went away. I quickly became immersed in traveling through China, taking in the local culture as we toured several universities. We returned in the middle of August. I was generally healthy, although I had been diagnosed with rheumatoid arthritis several years before. I would give myself injections in my thigh once a week. The medication left me feeling a little nauseous most of the time and commanded my focus. As such, I didn't think about the bump again.

A couple of months later, my wife and I were packing for our annual tradition of traveling to a University of Tennessee game and then going to the nearby mountains to celebrate our wedding anniversary. As we were driving up to Gatlinburg, my tongue brushed over something foreign that hurt. It was a bump in my mouth, similar to the one I had found in July. As I sat in the stands taking in the game, I started to wonder what this bump could be. *Is this something I need to worry about?* I thought. The cheering in the stadium quickly distracted me, and I shifted my focus to watching football. After the game, my wife and I drove over to enjoy the mountains for the rest of the weekend. I mentioned the bump to her, and we agreed that I should get it checked out. We enjoyed hiking and some fishing, although the bump was a constant reminder due to its location. Every time I ate or drank something, it would hurt. When we got back on Tuesday, October 20, I called my doctor's office. I explained that the bump had returned and scheduled an appointment for November 2.

When I arrived at my appointment, I explained when I noticed the bump and how I was feeling. My doctor examined me and said, "You know Bill, I still think this is a blocked salivary gland. However, let's be on the safe side and get it checked out. Come with me."

My doctor walked me down the hall and introduced me to his colleague, who was an ear, nose and throat (ENT) specialist. The office staff was able to fit me into his schedule after a short wait. He examined me and agreed that he thought it was a blocked salivary gland. He looked at me and said, "Let's be on the safe side and run some tests. Do you mind if I take a biopsy? I am going to have to cut your lip open." It seemed important, so I agreed. He numbed my lip before he took the sample. Numbing my lip hurt more than the biopsy. As he started to cut the skin, blood was spurting in several directions. Despite the mess, he was able to get the sample tissue and then stitched up my lip with four stitches. He said, "I'll send this off to the lab, and we'll find out what it is. We will be in touch soon." I thanked him and left the office, my lip a little sore from the procedure. Everything I ate and drank after the biopsy was a constant reminder of this bump as it stung and hurt when food or liquid brushed over it. After the stitches were taken out, I was able to forget about the bump and didn't think much about how long it was taking for the results.

I remember the next thing that happened related to this bump like it was yesterday. It was three weeks after the biopsy. My wife and I were grocery shopping in Publix on the day before Thanksgiving. We were preparing to host our family for the holiday. My wife was in front of me picking out sweet potatoes as I stood nearby with the shopping cart. My phone rang, and I noticed my doctor's name lighting up the face of the phone. I answered and heard, "Bill, I have the test results to share with you. I am so sorry to be calling you, as I would usually bring you in for a consultation like this, but the lab has been behind on processing the tissue. I am at the airport flying out to see my parents for Thanksgiving. I wanted you to have the long weekend to process what we learned." As I heard these words, my face turned white and my stomach became very queasy. I felt uneasy on my feet, like I was going to faint and was grateful that I was pushing the shopping cart, as it probably held me up. He said "I need to tell you—you have stage III-IV non-Hodgkin's lymphoma. I will refer you to an oncologist when I am back in the office on Monday." I stood there, frozen in my tracks, and lost touch with where I was for a minute. I took a deep breath and gathered my wits about me as we finished our shopping.

When my wife and I had loaded the groceries and gotten into my truck, she looked over at me and said, "Who was that on the phone?"

I turned to her and said, "It was my doctor. I've got cancer, and it's not good. It is the B-cell type and fast growing." I reached over and hugged her across the armrest, tears gushing from our eyes, as the words *cancer* permeated our minds. After we both ran out of tears, I looked at her and said, "I'm going to beat this. I'm not ready to leave you." As I looked around the bustling parking lot, I noticed people looking back at us, perhaps wondering, *What are those old people doing?* We had probably been sitting there for thirty minutes, taking up a parking space in the crowded lot. I started the car and drove home, while my wife called our daughter and asked her to meet us at the house. She pulled into our driveway just as we were driving down the street.

We went inside and shared the news as we all sat in the living room. Tears poured down our cheeks. After a while, I looked at them and said, "This is going to be a journey for all of us. We are going to beat this. I need y'all with me. We need to start praying now." When we finished praying, I closed my eyes and took in what I had just learned. *Cancer was spreading through my body. It was not just a clogged salivary gland. Wow. How could this happen?* I breathed in deeply and shifted my focus to survival and away from questioning, if not for me, then for my daughter and wife. I dug deep and imagined taking the next step toward climbing the tall mountain that I was facing. *I am going to beat this,* I thought.

We experienced one of the quietest Thanksgiving holidays ever as our lives had changed forever. Each of us went through the day feeling numb, still not believing the news and wanting it to go away. On Monday, my doctor's office called to say they had scheduled an appointment for the following week, on Thursday, with an oncologist who specializes in blood-borne cancers. The waiting was crippling at times as I fought with my mind, thinking *Why me?* and then racing forward to *What if?* My work and senate service helped distract me and keep my days full. It was finally Thursday, and I went to my appointment with my wife and my daughter. After discussing my history, the doctor said, "Based on the lab report, your type of cancer is called non-Hodgkin's lymphoma and it is between stage III and IV. We need to be aggressive in getting treatment started soon." *Wow, that sounds pretty serious all of a sudden*, I thought. He continued, "We will take some blood and run more tests. Then you will need to have a port-a-cath installed and have a procedure to take a sample from your lymph nodes. I know this is a lot of information. What questions do you have for me?"

I looked at him, a little in disbelief at the words that had just come out of his mouth. As I held my wife's hand, I took a deep breath and felt his words permeate through my mind—I have stage III–IV cancer. I asked him some clarifying questions about the next steps. Information felt like power in this moment, and we had next steps. *I can move forward now. I am determined to beat this cancer*, I thought.

I went in for the lymph node procedure at the hospital a week later with a Correct Chemo™ kit in my hand. Vanderbilt University had been using this predictive test kit for the past eight years with cancer patients. Based on a tissue sample from an individual, the test reveals which chemotherapy agent, or combination of agents, will kill the cancer cells of a specific patient. I handed the kit to the nurse, and she gave me a puzzled look, then went to get the doctor. This predictive test was still considered experimental, and the surgeon questioned its use. He was not sure if he would be able to get enough tissue from the lymph node for both tests. I felt he was resisting because he would not get paid extra for this test, although he was already getting paid to perform the procedure, and it didn't require any extra effort. I pushed back hard and insisted that he get a sample for the kit. I was going to find a surgeon who would perform this test, as I wanted to give myself the highest chances of survival. He finally acquiesced and was able to get enough tissue for both purposes.

While I was going through this series of steps to inform my treatment plan, my mother's health continued to deteriorate. She was living in a nursing home, and it was clear she was nearing the end of her life. The night before I went in to have my port-a-cath installed, our whole family gathered in my mom's room. *The Sound of Music* was on television. We watched the movie and enjoyed singing along to the songs with Julie Andrews—songs like "My Favorite Things" and "Do-Re-Mi"—while my mother slept. I had not told her about my cancer, although we were talking about it in the room. We all decided to sleep in her room with her that night, wanting to be with her and have her feel our love until the end. The next morning, I said good-bye to her, and my wife took me to my procedure. When I came out of the procedure and was in recovery, my wife let me know that my mother had died. I was still groggy from the anesthesia, although I understood what she had said. I started sobbing uncontrollably. Here I was facing cancer treatment, and now I would be walking through the grief of losing my mother at the same time. I closed my eyes and said a prayer. It was time to reach down deeper into my soul and grab more strength to somehow to face my grief and my treatment at the same time.

Treatment Experience

The report from the Correct Chemo™ predictive test came back with the recommended types of chemotherapy that would kill the cancer. I shared it with my doctor, and he decided to follow the recommended drug therapy, which was Rubex and Doxil, known as Red Devil. "This is not going to beat me," was my mantra for the four months of chemotherapy. I went in for my first infusion the first week of January. Red Devil is a very lethal drug, and other drugs are used in combination to help with the process. For me, the nurse started with an IV bag of Benadryl every time. It would expand my blood vessels and increase the ability for the chemo drug to permeate my veins. My daughter came with me to every infusion. She worked for our family insurance business and was able to take more time away than my wife, who also worked full time. Once the nurse started the IV drip of Benadryl, I would pass out cold for about an hour. While I was asleep, I started hallucinating from the drug and was unaware of what I was doing. The woman in the chair next to me had her arm on the arm rest. I started patting her arm, thinking it was a dog. Laughter in the room startled me, and I woke me up and heard from my daughter what I had done. It was helpful to have some humor in the midst of the process, which was trying for all of us.

While I was undergoing chemotherapy treatment, the legislature was in session. I took my role representing my community very seriously. I was not willing to let my constituents down or disappoint anyone during the session, although I imagine they would have understood. I was determined to keep working and never missed a vote. I had a couch in my office and would come back to sleep during committee breaks. My stomach always felt queasy. I would sleep in my suit on the couch and wake up in a full sweat. Staying focused on the legislative session was a useful distraction, which kept me focused on something other than my cancer and my grief from losing my mom. The session enabled me to focus on something greater than myself, which kept me from feeling sorry for myself about my condition.

I experienced many of the common side effects of chemotherapy, including severe diarrhea, nausea, night sweats, vomiting, chills, and hiccups that wouldn't stop. I was convinced that I would be the one patient not to lose my hair. I was showering one morning a week after the first infusion, and as I was shampooing my hair, clumps of it came out and fell in my face. *Oh crap, here we go,* I thought. It kept coming out as I finished my shower. I stepped onto the bathmat as I toweled off, looking in the mirror. The visual I saw is still etched in my memory—I looked like I had mange, the skin disease caused by parasitic mites. This was the first visible side effect I had experienced. I swallowed several times as I continued to look in the mirror, feeling vulnerable and humble. I had seen people in the grocery store with hair like this before; empathy grew inside of me for how they must have felt. I looked down at my watch and noticed the time. I needed to get to my office soon for a meeting, and I stopped at Starbucks on my way and ordered a coffee. As I pulled up to the drive-through window, the barista smiled as she turned toward me with the coffee. She took a second look, turned away and turned back, as if to make sure of what she was seeing. Her facial expression turned from a smile to one of concern, and she held her hand way out to give me my coffee and change. Her gesture made me feel like she was worried about catching whatever I had if she got too close, as if I was contagious. Here was my first experience of the physical signs of cancer bringing out interesting responses in others, and it would not be my last—a constant reminder that I was sick.

Hiccups were the most annoying of my symptoms, as they would not stop. I tried several home remedies with no luck. My brother-in-law recommended a trick he had learned while serving as a medic in Vietnam. I was willing to try anything at this point. He told me to take the head off a cross pen, put it inside my ear right in the middle and press down. I think there must be a nerve in there, as it would stop the hiccups. I experienced excruciating pain in my bones throughout treatment. I tried taking a pain pill just once. It made me loopy and dizzy, but I still felt the pain. While many cancer patients lose weight on chemotherapy, I gained almost fifteen pounds, probably a side effect of the steroids I was taking. My hair turned white during the treatment, but later grew back in my natural color.

I was so touched by all the friends and constituents who showed me such support and compassion, too many to recount here. One of the most memorable was a card I received every week from a Sunday school class of women in my district. The card said that they were praying for me and lifting me up every day. Every one of them personally signed each card. I grew to look forward to receiving this card, as it gave me such energy to persevere. My secretary's husband had participated in a mission trip to Africa the year before and had met a prayer group of women. When he learned about my cancer, he tracked them down through email and requested that they add me to their prayer list. Another memorable experience was when I was invited to have lunch at local churches. People would read the Bible to me and then rub healing oil on my forehead. Given the advanced nature of my cancer, I was open to experiencing new ways of healing and felt these events were orchestrated by God. I felt supported by the entire community I served, as if each constituent was making a difference in my healing each day. The outpouring of support touched every cell of my body in a loving way.

When the legislative session was over at the end of May, I had completed chemotherapy, and it was time for another PET scan. I went to the hospital in the morning for the scan, and then arrived at my doctor's office that afternoon to hear the results. With my wife and daughter at my side, I heard something I wasn't expecting. The doctor looked at me and said, "Bill, I am sorry to say the treatment didn't work. Your cancer is now full stage IV."

I felt deflated, as if all the air had been released from a balloon. I asked quietly, "What are my options?" I was still in shock from the news.

He said, "We can try stem cell replacement therapy. That is really our only option since the chemotherapy didn't work."

I swallowed a couple of times and asked what would happen next as I gathered strength I didn't know I had.

He said, "We are going to have to take some bone marrow from your pelvis to see if you can accept your own." Stem cell transplants are used to replace bone marrow that has been destroyed by cancer or by the chemotherapy used to treat the cancer.

I asked, "What happens if I'm not a match?"

The room got even quieter as he paused before replying. He explained that if I was not a match, I would have to wait until they found a donor, which could take some time. He outlined the next steps, and we left the office. Time was not something I had an abundance of at this point, with stage IV cancer spreading through my body. As we drove home, tears poured down our cheeks, not knowing what the next step would bring.

Once we were home, I closed my eyes and processed what he had said. *I am staring death in the face*, I thought. *Wow, okay God, if it is my time to go, take me now.* In our human condition, some of us live life with a false sense of being in control of what might happen next or that tomorrow will come just like today did. Here I was, facing the great unknown and feeling totally at the mercy of God. My wife, daughter, and I gathered together and prayed, asking for guidance during the process and grace to be able to endure the highs and lows. Our prayers were answered when I learned that I would be able to accept my own stem cells in the transplant process. With this news, we were able to take another step forward in the treatment plan.

A few days later, my wife and I attended an all-day education session to learn about stem cell replacement: the process, the challenges, and how very tenuous life would become with a compromised immune system. It was a little overwhelming, and I found myself shifting my focus to work during the day. The next day, I went back to the hospital to have a Trifusion catheter implanted on my left side near my heart for the transplant process. Since I still had the port-a-cath on my right side from the chemotherapy, I looked like I was deformed—two sets of nipples were protruding from my shirt. While I am not a vain person, my strange looking chest really messed with my mind. I learned to get used to strange looks from people in the parking lot.

The senators I served with knew about my cancer. One of them had had stem cell treatment before and recounted her experience. She had not used the pain medication they offered. Medical advancements in stem cell replacement had recently yielded a new machine that enabled harvesting of the stem cells by punching through the pelvis, which was a much less invasive procedure.

I went into the hospital for the procedure, and as they were preparing me, the doctor asked if I wanted any morphine. I thought back to my fellow colleague's story and, trying to be tough, I said, "No thank you." I started to rethink my answer while the technician inserted the machine in my hip and a bone-crunching sound permeated the room. I was lying on my stomach and felt my entire body lift off the table; it was the most excruciating pain I had ever felt. The technician then used a device that looked similar to a turkey baster to start sucking the bone marrow out of my hip. When he was finished, I looked over at him and asked, "Why did it hurt so much?" The technician explained that my blood was thin and shot out fast, like a geyser. He imagined that my colleague's blood was thicker and flowed more slowly. *Oh great, next time I will opt for pain medicine, if there is a next time,* I thought. The plan was to harvest five million stem cells, but they were only able to get three million, so I was to come back the next morning for another round.

When I arrived home after the procedure, I had a very odd feeling, like I had swallowed the sun. I felt a rush from the tips of my toes all the way up to the hairs on my head. I looked at my wife and said, "Honey, I think I am having a hot flash."

She looked at me, smiled, and said, "Yes, don't you remember hearing about that in the training?"

I said, "Well, I thought they were talking about women, not men. Guess I wasn't paying attention." Evidently, one of the side effects of harvesting stem cells in men is it can trigger menopausal symptoms.

I was more prepared on day two of this process, thinking it would be my last. I asked for the pain medication. My daughter had let me borrow her ear buds, and I had my iPad with me, ready to listen to *Hotel California* loud enough that I would not hear the bone crunch. When my doctor came in about nine o'clock, I turned to him and said, "Doctor, I have a question. My wife told me that harvesting the stem cells could trigger menopause in men. Is that true? I only have one female gene and it enables me to pick out my clothes. I can't have any more of this."

He started chuckling and said, "You've got one female gene, really? I hope you will still be able to pick out your clothes after this." We both laughed, and it lightened the mood. Humor helped shift how I felt, allowing me to focus on something other than the treatment I was enduring. The technician completed the process, this time without my hearing the bone crunching and without feeling pain. When all was finished, I learned that I would have to come back the next day for a third time, as they still didn't have the five million stem cells they needed. I was becoming practiced in an experience that was potentially life-giving, although not something I would have opted for under normal circumstances.

During the time between the procedures, I experienced an empty feeling in the pit of my stomach, wondering what the outcome of this treatment would be. I was imagining my full life and wondering what it would be like without me in it, worrying about my family, my work, and my friends and how they would manage. Would I be able to see my daughter get married? Just as the thoughts popped into my head, distractions from work or life would shift my focus back to surviving. *I am going to beat this!* Once I knew that the third procedure had yielded all the required stem cells, I was given a day off to get my affairs in order before the replacement process started. I then checked into the hospital for the conditioning phase. When I was in my room, the doctor explained that they were going to pump my body with the strongest chemotherapy ever. The goal was to damage and possibly destroy my bone marrow during conditioning. The nurse would come in my room every day to run tests to gauge the level of my immune system, waiting for the moment when there was none. After six days, I was given another day off, although I was in a highly sterilized environment, so it wasn't like I could go fishing. I slept most of the day. The next day, the doctor came back with my stem cells for the transplant process. The nurse warmed them up and then hooked me up to the machine to pump them into my body through the Trifusion port. I looked a little like a squid with three different tubes hanging out, each four inches long. I stayed in the hospital for a few days for observation and was then released home with instructions. The nurse said, "Two things may happen after you go home. You may get severe diarrhea, or you may get a fever of 100.2 degrees. If either of these happens, you have one hour to get back to the hospital."

I lived thirty minutes away, which made the ability to return within the hour window possible. On day two, my fever started to increase. When it reached 100.2, my wife called the ER and the doctor to let them know we were on our way. The doctor had given me a VIP card that would enable me to go into the back of the ER and bypass registration. Just after getting in the back door, I started throwing up. I was checked into the hospital again with heavy antibiotics for ten days. I wondered why I had been discharged the first time. I looked at my doctor and asked, "Why did you send me home? And what is the percentage of time that either one of these two outcomes happen following the transplant process?"

He looked at me, grinned, and said, "The chance of either outcome happening is 82 percent. You are in the insurance business, right? The insurance company is taking a chance that you are one of the 18 percent who does not experience these side effects."

While in the hospital, I was required to be in an isolation room due to my compromised immune system. Every day, the nurse would come take blood. I was given two shots of Neupogen in my stomach to reduce the risk of infection. I later learned that each shot cost around $5,000. During this period in isolation, I slept most of the time and watched television when I had some energy. I had just about enough energy to go to the bathroom. Every day, food service brought in meals for me, although I still wasn't able to taste food, nor was I able to smell anything. I also had developed neuropathy in my toes. Even with these longer-lasting side effects, I felt grateful, as they beat the alternative of dying.

I was discharged after thirty days. I focused every day on gaining strength, one breath at a time, one step at a time, as I healed from this strenuous process. I slowly added back normal activities and eventually was able to work again. I did change certain things in my life—I stopped smoking cigars and started exercising again, to name a couple. After ninety days, I went to a follow-up appointment with my doctor, along with my wife and daughter. The doctor opened the exam room door smiling, which was the surprise I'd been hoping for. He said, "Bill, you are in remission. There is no sign of the cancer."

I leapt off the table and hugged him, as my wife and daughter followed behind me, wrapping their arms around us. I pulled back to look at him and said, "Oh my goodness, what fantastic news! Thank you so much for sticking with me through all of this, it paid off!" It remains one of the most memorable days in my life. As I unpacked the meaning of each word he had said in my mind, I thanked God for saving me and decided he has more work for me to do here.

Advice for Others

How I supported myself
- Prayed daily.
- Kept working through treatment, a helpful distraction.
- Found humor in small things to lighten my mood.
- Had my wife and/or daughter at every appointment.
- Took deep belly breaths several times a day.

How others supported me
- Prayers from all over the world.
- Thoughtful cards, calls, and texts.
- Incredibly humble and compassionate care team through each step.

Helpful tips

- Don't sweat the small stuff, focus on the big picture.
- When something like this happens, take it as an opportunity to serve others with validation if they are going through a similar experience.
- Cancer hates oxygen—take the biggest deep breaths you can.
- Learn more about stem cell transplantation—it is a viable option in some cases.

DANA'S STORY

———— • ● • ————

It was the middle of September 2008 when I first noticed my back aching, right in the middle where it was hard to reach with my arm. It was a Sunday, and I thought I had just pulled a muscle moving some tables on the deck for a football party the day before. The pain had gone away by the next day, so I dismissed it as nothing. My youngest daughter was playing soccer at the time. When I would go watch her play at some away games at smaller schools that didn't have bleachers, I would stand for the hour and a half game. I started to notice my back aching again, and again I dismissed it as a pulled muscle. On Halloween, I went to see a horror movie with my husband. When I went to sit down in the chair, I felt some aching pain in my back and was not able to comfortably sit in the theater chair. I went up to the back of the theater and stood to watch the movie. The next day, I didn't feel the pain at all.

When I did feel the pain, it was an aching, gnawing pain similar to tooth pain, something I could tolerate. I started to wonder if maybe one of the discs in my spine was damaged. I was updating my husband, who is a doctor, about my pain the next day. He ordered some blood tests and an X-ray. The results came back normal, not showing any sign of an issue. While the test results came back normal, the pain continued to flare up and would increase as each day passed. I was continuing my normal activities and going to work, although I didn't feel up to exercising. When I was not able to walk anymore, my husband called a colleague who was a doctor of osteopathy (DO) and scheduled an appointment for me for the following day.

I went in for my appointment and explained the symptoms I was experiencing and when the pain would flare up. He examined me and then manipulated my back some, which caused pain spasms up and down my spine. He prescribed Darvocet for the pain and recommended an MRI, which he was able to schedule for later that evening. I left the office, picked up my prescription, and headed home. The pain was bad enough that I took one of the pills. It was the first time I had ever taken pain medication that strong, and I didn't know what to expect. I started to feel out of it, and my brain was not quite connecting normally. I would go to do something and forget what I was doing. When my husband came home from work, we ate dinner quickly and then he took me for the MRI. As I went to lie down on the narrow bed of the MRI machine, I felt a sharp pain and said, "I can't do this." I sat back up.

My husband asked, "Do you want me to stay in the room with you?" I told him yes, so he walked over next to me and held my foot for the procedure while the bed moved back under the magnet. The technician finished the MRI and then said he needed to do it one more time, this time with dye to show contrast. I was still not thinking clearly and didn't think much of this additional test. I did notice that my husband seemed to become more stoic and quieter, something he does when he is concerned.

When the technician finished the MRI, I got up and went to change back into my clothes. As I was walking back into the room, still feeling out of it from the pain medicine, I saw my husband talking to the radiologist, who had just read my MRI. I overheard him say, "I'm really sorry." My husband turned around and saw me and stopped talking to the radiologist.

We said good-bye and walked to the car holding hands. It was a cold evening and rain was pouring like buckets from the sky. As my husband drove us home, I looked over at him and said, "What is wrong with me?"

He looked straight ahead and in a quiet voice said, "We don't know yet."

I asked, "Do you think it's something bad?" I was watching him as he considered how to answer. He was brief in his response and said it might be bad. My mind was still groggy from the pain medication, and at that point, "something bad" in my mind was an issue with one of my discs.

The next day, November 12, my husband went to work, and I decided to stay home. I was getting more frustrated as the pain and discomfort continued to escalate. I am a planner and just wanted to know what was going on in my body so I could move forward. I really didn't like the way I had felt on the pain medication the night before, so I skipped taking one that morning. I decided to use the heating pad every few hours to manage the pain. My phone started to ring, and I noticed it was my doctor's office, probably with the MRI results. I answered the phone and heard, "Hi, Dana, don't worry, I haven't lost a lymphoma patient yet."

I sat in my chair in disbelief of what he had just said. I asked, "Do I have lymphoma?" I was sitting there waiting for a response for what felt like minutes.

Then he said, "Oh my God, I thought you already knew. Oh, Dana, I am so sorry. Yes, you do have lymphoma. The MRI showed a tumor on your spinal cord. We will move quickly and get you in for more tests. I will be back in touch soon with more details. Hang in there." I hung up and stared at the phone, trying to sort out in my mind the words I had just heard. My thoughts shifted to my husband and why he hadn't told me. I started to imagine that if my husband had been the one to say those words to me, he would have completely broken down. As a doctor, he knew too much about medical conditions and chances for survival. And in reality,

I knew that he did not want to be the one to tell his wife that she had cancer.

I called my husband and asked him to come home, then called my mother and asked her to come over. My mom had been diagnosed early in 2008 with liver disease. She was managing pretty well with medication and watching her diet. My mom arrived first, and as I shared the news with her, she quickly reached out and wrapped her arms around me. She held me for a while, and although the word "cancer" was still permeating through my mind, I remained positive, never imagining that I would not survive. My husband arrived soon after and asked me what the doctor had said. As the three of us sat there discussing what was going on, I remember not thinking much of it. We were talking in a matter-of-fact way, like I had the flu or something much more innocuous than cancer.

The toughest conversation I had was with my seventeen-year-old daughter, who was a junior in high school. I wanted to protect her and make sure she would be okay. When she arrived home later that day, I told her I had some news to share with her. She and I sat on the couch in the living room, just the two of us, as I said, "Remember that pain I have been having in my back? I found out today it is cancer. I promise I will fight with everything I have to beat it. I am comfortable with you being as involved as you want to be. I love you." Tears streamed down both of our cheeks as I leaned over to hug her. I shared more details about what would happen next, and we made a plan for dinner. After she went up to her room to do homework, I called the vice principal. I wanted him to know what was going on so the school could support her. I also requested that she be able to attend as many of my appointments and treatments as she wanted. He was kind and compassionate in his response and gave his approval for her to miss school. My husband called our older daughter, who was away at college, and shared the news with her.

My doctor ordered additional pre-cancer treatment studies fairly quickly, including a biopsy and a CT scan scheduled for the following week. I filed for a medical leave of absence and stopped working. If I had been examined independently, the other lymph nodes in my neck and abdomen were not yet large enough to indicate something was wrong. The tumor on my spinal cord was the indication that something was wrong, which did not show on the X-ray but did on the MRI. I believe that if that tumor was not where it was causing the pain, I would not have known for a longer time and my situation likely would have been worse and very different. This tumor was my saving grace and led me to get it checked out. On November 19, I went to the hospital for more tests with my husband. They drew blood and then prepared me for the biopsy, which was completed through a lumbar puncture.

My appointment with the oncologist had been scheduled the same day, after the tests. I remember walking into his office with my husband. He was sitting at his desk wearing a purple shirt. He was an older gentleman and was talking about his retirement as he stood up to walk toward me. He pulled up a chair in front of me, scooted forward until his knees were touching mine, and looked me in the eye. In that moment, as I was preparing my mind to talk about treatment with him, the reality of my condition and the emotion of what that meant caught up to me. Tears started pouring down my cheeks. He knew what I was facing and handled my emotions with grace and compassion. He explained the options I had for treatment, including surgically removing the tumor. I was not interested in back surgery and said no thank you. He had been able to see the results from the biopsy and explained my diagnosis, non-Hodgkin's lymphoma. Then he started to explain his plan for chemotherapy and radiation. I didn't even think about asking what stage the cancer was. I believed I would survive, and ignorance felt like bliss to me at that point.

"Dana, we are going to start you on radiation, five days a week, for four weeks. Then we will use a chemotherapy drug regimen known as R-Chop, which is a combination of four drugs and an antibody. We have had great results with this regimen for people with lymphoma. We are going to start your chemo infusions soon after you start the radiation treatments, and you will have seven infusions, one every three weeks. The downside is, you are likely to lose your hair." What registered most in those words I heard was, *My hair, I am going to lose my hair! Oh no, I love my thick hair.* That was the moment when the full reality sunk in as I imagined the physical side effects of the cancer treatment starting to show. I started sobbing uncontrollably. My husband put his arms around me as I fell apart. He told me that he would be with me every step of the way, and would oversee my treatment plan, which gave me comfort. I trusted him both as my husband and as a doctor and felt grateful for his love and expertise given my diagnosis.

Treatment Experience

I was able to start radiation the next day and completed seven rounds and one chemotherapy infusion by Thanksgiving, when my older daughter came home from college. The radiation made me extremely tired, and the prednisone kept me awake at night; it was a tough combination to be tired and unable to sleep! My daughters and I went to have a pedicure together on Sunday after Thanksgiving. It felt good to keep somewhat of a normal routine and be able to catch up on what was going on in their lives, a welcome distraction from my cancer treatment. We went to a salon where we had been many times before. In the process of completing my pedicure, the nail technician somehow cut my big toe. It hurt, though it seemed minor compared to the treatment I was enduring. Two days later on Tuesday, I woke up with a 105-degree fever. I felt horrible and asked my youngest daughter to drive me to my radiation appointment. When I arrived and the nurse took my temperature, she said, "You have a high fever. I am going to call your doctor. I'll be right back." Because of my condition and the stage of my cancer, the next thing I knew I was being admitted to the hospital. I learned that I had an infection that was causing the high fever. I spent six days in the hospital, with IV antibiotics flowing through my veins. While I was in the hospital, I was wheeled down for a lumbar puncture to be sure there were no cancer cells in my spinal fluid given that the tumor was on my spinal cord at T8–9. On day six, my doctor came by to let me know that I would be able to go home. He also shared that I didn't need any more radiation treatments, as the radiation had shrunk the tumor so much it was no longer visible.

I didn't know for months what stage my cancer had advanced to. It seemed unimportant in the beginning. When I would think about my diagnosis and the situation, I would think, *My daughter is only seventeen, and I haven't gone on a honeymoon yet. I am not going to die; I still have much to do in my life.* Throughout the period of learning of my diagnosis and completing my treatment, I had faith that I would push through it. I would keep doing what my husband and my doctor recommended so it would all end well. Eventually I found out my cancer was stage IV. I retained a lot of fluid and felt puffy during treatment due to the steroids, so I wore sweats most of the time. While off work, I would welcome friends and family for visits, although I didn't feel comfortable seeing anyone from work. It was a personal experience, and I felt at my worst.

When my hair started to fall out, I cried again. I loved my thick hair, and this was a visible sign that I was sick. I decided to cut my hair short and thought that would work, that no one would notice. I kept my normal routine of getting a manicure every Saturday. My mom would come wash my hair and blow it out, which helped me feel some semblance of normal life. A couple of months later, I was in the hospital where I worked and riding the elevator up to my office, which was one floor above the oncology floor. I stopped at the oncology floor and a man got in. He looked at me and said, "Oh, you must have cancer. So do I." I realized then that my trick of wearing short hair was not fooling anyone and decided to shave my head. It was so humbling to face this step, having to let go of something that I loved, something that made me feel like myself. The treatment really zapped my energy, and I had a hard time doing much of anything. *I am never going to be normal again*, I thought. I was most disheartened by losing my hair, not only on my head but also on my arms and legs. It was really unsettling to me. I wore scarves on my head to minimize the shock of my new bald look. I could tell how uncomfortable my baldness was for others in public places by the look on their faces. I could tell by their reaction how it freaked them out when I would talk to them. My daughter had finished soccer and was now participating in competitive cheerleading. I was able to make it to every competition except for one, which was a weekend tournament in Indianapolis. Throughout my treatment, I had strived to limit the impact of my cancer treatment on my younger daughter, who still lived at home. My daughter was really upset, and I felt relieved to hear that my older daughter was able to travel to Indianapolis for the competition.

While my family was my rock and unconditional support through my treatment, the most impactful part of my healing was God. I could feel His presence at different times. I am convinced that my faith was instrumental and foundational to surviving such a late-stage cancer diagnosis. I would pray and ask for guidance, saying things like, "Show me what You want me to do with this. I realize You can work wonders, show me how." Following the end of my chemotherapy in late March 2009, my doctor ordered blood work and a PET scan to make sure the cancer was gone. In August of 2009, I had the same tests repeated and learned I was in remission. I breathed a big sigh of relief and knew that God had guided every step of my healing. My mom supported me through all of my treatment, despite her health condition. I felt so loved and cared for by her and my whole family.

While I was living this experience, through the highs and lows of enduring cancer treatment and the many side effects, I thought I was never going to feel better. And then one day I did. Where I sit today, I realize the experience has changed me for the better. I stopped putting work first and have made more time for myself and for friendships. I started eating healthier and living life to its fullest, not putting off until tomorrow what could be done today. At a recent annual physical, my doctor said, "This is the best I have seen your blood work, ever." I attribute my remission eleven years later, despite a stage IV cancer diagnosis, to my husband, my daughters, my family, my faith, and my positive outlook on life.

Since going through my cancer journey, I have been a volunteer with the Leukemia and Lymphoma Society (LSS) in several capacities. Light the Night is their biggest fund raiser, and I've participated and raised money with a walk team every year since 2009 and served on the walk executive committee both in Pennsylvania and here in Nashville. The most meaningful volunteering that I do with LLS, however, is as a First Connection volunteer. I am connected to newly diagnosed patients to listen, answer questions, and share my journey as someone who has been there. My hope is that I am able to help others hold on to hope as they face fighting cancer.

Advice for Others

How I supported myself

- I had a calendar to keep track of doctor appointments and treatments.
- I prayed and talked to God.
- I trusted my husband's recommendations for my treatment.
- I took a break from work.
- I would go to the salon at eight o'clock before they opened for a weekly manicure.
- Being able to greet my daughter when she came home from school every day expanded my heart, as it was the first time ever since I worked outside of the home.

How others supported me

- My friends and family called to check on me and sent many cards, which I posted on my bulletin board.
- We had lots of meals delivered, which really helped.
- Friends helped me decorate for holidays.
- Friends would come visit me during my chemotherapy infusions.

Helpful tips

- Engage with your friends, acquaintances, or loved ones when you learn of their diagnosis; fear is so powerful—don't be afraid to say you care.
- Acknowledge the situation—including saying you have no words if that is the case, or say, "I heard something about you that makes me sad or worried about you, you are in my thoughts and prayers;" know that withdrawing feels hurtful to the cancer patient.
- When you learn of an immune system-based cancer diagnosis, such as non-Hodgkin's lymphoma, know that you are putting the patient at risk if you hug them or shake their hand.
- If you want to help, organize a meal train or go buy house staples such as drinks, Tupperware, toilet paper, and paper towels; just drop them on the porch and let the person know, as it can be overwhelming to the cancer patient to tell you what they need.
- Every single cancer experience is unique: Be thoughtful about saying things like "I understand how you feel" or "I know what you are going through," even if you are a survivor.
- Offer to drive children to activities, school, or appointments.
- Keep your commitments—if you say you are going to stop by at a certain time, do it.

BILL G'S STORY

———— • ● • ————

It was the summer of 1979, and I was a thirty-three-year-old father of three girls, all under the age of ten. When I would look in the mirror in the morning to brush my teeth, I started to notice two small lumps on either side of my neck. *Maybe they are pimples, probably nothing to be concerned about*, I thought. When they didn't go away, I thought perhaps I was having an allergic reaction to something and started putting topical cream on them. When the lumps were still there after a few months, I became a little concerned. I am a fairly vain person and was acutely aware of the impact the lumps had on my appearance. I worked in sales and thought my looks mattered a lot. My wife did not work outside of the home at the time. We were both focused on raising our children and keeping up with the busyness of life, and these lumps stayed in the background of our focus. A few months later, I made an appointment with my primary care physician. When my doctor walked into the exam room, he asked about my symptoms and then examined me. He said, "I can't really determine anything by looking at the lumps. I think you need to go to a surgeon. I am happy to refer you if that would be helpful." I thanked him and graciously declined his offer for a referral. Then I called my brother-in-law, who was an internist.

I explained what was going on, and he referred me to a general surgeon, one he recommended highly.

I was able to schedule an appointment in a few days, probably because of my brother-in-law's referral. When the surgeon came in the exam room, he examined me and said, "Bill, this is not a serious operation, although I am going to have to get these taken out. The lumps are under the skin, so it will have to be performed in surgery." *Surgery, wow what a surprise. I am not experiencing any symptoms of anything being wrong,* I thought. The surgeon explained what would happen next and scheduled the surgery, which would be done in the office under local anesthesia, for the following week. I went on with my life and quickly dismissed it as nothing to worry about.

I showed up to the surgeon's office, and he performed the procedure under local anesthesia. A week later, I went back to see the surgeon to get my stitches removed. When he came into the exam room, he said, "Bill, I need to refer you to a hematologist."

I was startled and said, "You've got to be kidding me! That's a blood doctor, isn't it?" *That was the last thing I expected to hear.* I thought back to my appointment and did not recall him saying that he would be sending a sample of the lump tissue out for tests.

He said, "You have some type of cancer." I sat there in complete disbelief. He could have knocked me off the chair with a feather in that moment. I kept staring at the wall and then back at him, completely stunned. My family flashed before my eyes: here I was, a young man with three young daughters, and now I have cancer? *There must be some mistake,* I thought. After a period of uncomfortable silence, he added, "Bill, you've got to get this evaluated further. You have a form of cancer, which is all I know right now." Most everything in my life I had wanted to be positive, until I faced this biopsy result, which I had wanted to be negative. I was not remotely prepared to hear I had cancer.

I told the surgeon that I wanted to call my brother-in-law while I was there. I was able to get him on the phone and have him talk to the surgeon. I was still in complete disbelief that I had cancer. The surgeon explained a few things to my brother-in-law, and then put me back on the phone. He said, "Bill I am going to suggest you go see this specific specialist I know who is a hematologist–oncologist. He will be able to gather more information for you." I walked out of the office in a fog, not really aware of my surroundings. Somehow, I managed to find my car, and when I got in, I thought about what I had just heard again. *I have cancer.* The words kept ringing in my ears. I had thought this was going to be a simple appointment to get my stitches removed and was planning to go back to work. *On second thought, I better go home and tell my wife.* I drove home and found my wife in the kitchen, preparing dinner. I said, "Hey, I just had my stitches removed at the doctor's office. I need to talk to you about something he said. As you know, he took the lumps out." At this point, my wife stopped chopping the vegetables and turned to look at me. I continued, "I didn't realize they were going to test the lumps. The tests came back positive, and I have some form of cancer."

An uncomfortable silence filled the room for what felt like five minutes. Then she said, in a concerned voice, "So what are you going to do next?" I explained that my brother-in-law had given me the name of a hematologist–oncologist, and I needed to go see him to learn more. I added, "As a matter of fact, I think we both need to go." She agreed and said I'd better get an appointment soon. About that time, my phone rang. My brother-in-law had called the specialist and was able to schedule an appointment in a few days, likely because of his relationship.

My life was changing by the moment, and I walked around a little dazed, still sorting out my new reality. I managed to make it through the next few days with the distraction of work and taking care of our girls. My wife and I arrived at the appointment and met the specialist. He looked at me and said, "Based on initial test results from your surgery, you have some form of lymphoma."

I looked at him puzzled and said, "What's that?" He explained that it was a blood-based type of cancer that affects the lymphatic system. As I sat there trying to make sense of his words, I started to wonder, *What did I do to get this? Was the mononucleosis I had in high school to blame?* The specialist said it was not likely related and wasn't sure how I had gotten cancer. He explained that he would need to run more tests, and his nurse would be in shortly to draw blood. Then, we would come back and meet with him in a few days. I scheduled an appointment for three days later, and I left to focus on our girls and my work.

On a warm summer day a few days later, my wife and I arrived at the follow-up appointment. When the doctor came in the room, he looked at me with a calm and caring expression and said, "Bill, the type of cancer you have is called non-Hodgkin's lymphoma. It is stage I. You will need to undergo treatment that includes chemotherapy and radiation." I felt comforted by his presence and how he talked to me, which helped me relax a little. My new reality of being a cancer patient was settling in, and I felt like I could trust this doctor.

The next thing that happened completely shocked me. My wife spoke up and said, "How long is Bill going to live?"

The doctor was startled by the question and replied, "Well, I actually don't know; it could be two years or ten years or more."

She gave him a determined look and said, "I need to know."

The doctor looked at me, and I looked at him, completely not believing what we were hearing. After an uncomfortable silence, the doctor said, "I wouldn't go there now, because there are a lot of things we can do to treat this."

The next thing she said was, "Why me?" *Did I really just hear those words come out of her mouth? I'm the one with the cancer,* I thought. I gave her a puzzled look, attempting to signal to her that what she had said may not have come out as she intended.

The doctor watched this interchange between my wife and me and didn't say anything. I imagine doctors hear all kinds of comments in difficult situations like ours. He may not have thought too much of it, but it completely stunned me. After a few minutes, he looked at her and said, "We have a ways to go. We are going to start some chemotherapy on Bill to try to get this cancer under control."

The thought of not surviving had not crossed my mind yet. Now the subject of death was on the table, front and center, after what my wife had said. I left the office distressed, not only by my diagnosis, but by my wife's reaction to it. I wasn't sure which one troubled me most. My wife was a really smart woman, very matter-of-fact in her interactions, and she wanted to know the facts. She was driven and organized, but not very warm. As I thought about it more on our silent drive home, I realized that her reaction didn't overly surprise me.

When we got home, she said, "What are we going to do about it?"

I looked at her, puzzled, and said, "What do you mean? We are going to do what every other cancer patient does. I am going to go through chemotherapy and radiation and hope for the best." I was able to be calm in my response, although I was still sorting it all out. We talked about the children and decided not to tell them yet. I wasn't ready to share the news with anyone else at this point, except people who needed to know. My brother-in-law knew, and I needed to tell my manager at work. When I called my manager, I said, "I have been diagnosed with cancer. I don't know what's going to happen with the business while I'm undergoing treatment, but I'm going to focus on getting this cancer under control." I knew that was a bold statement to make to my manager, although it was how I felt.

He replied, "Bill, don't even worry about the business. This sounds serious. Go and get well."

Treatment Experience

My doctor arranged for the treatment to start soon. I was to have chemotherapy infusions once a week for thirteen weeks and then radiation once a week for fifteen weeks. The following week, on a Friday, I drove myself to the hospital for my first chemotherapy infusion. The chemotherapy drug regimen he used is known as R-Chop, which is a combination of four drugs and an antibody. I had called before driving over to make sure I would be able to drive. As I walked into the waiting room, a very awkward feeling permeated every cell in my body. I saw several men who were completely bald and several women wearing scarves on their heads. It was one of the most uncomfortable situations I had ever experienced. I am not usually someone who is unable to find words, although in this moment, I was speechless. *Oh my God, this is real,* I thought. When I was called back for my infusion, there were two other people sitting in chairs getting treatment. The whole process took about three hours. I was still in shock from my observations in the waiting room. I only talked to the nurses and kept to myself while I did some work. I had brought my cell phone to the appointment and made some calls during the three hours. I went home after the treatment and had a normal evening, although the scene I had experienced was etched in my memory. The next day, I went outside to cut the grass, something I did every Saturday. I was trying to maintain my normal activities and didn't want to disappoint my wife. I was concerned about worrying her with one more thing to do. As I was mowing the grass, I could feel my energy drain out of my toes as if someone had pulled a plug in my feet. I was able to finish mowing and go inside to shower. Then I fell into bed, fully exhausted.

Sundays were my night to cook dinner for our family. It was a fun tradition that I really enjoyed. On Saturday afternoon, I was looking through a cookbook to choose what I was going to make the next night. I fell asleep in the chair, with the recipe book in hand. My wife came and woke me up. She was seeing the impact of the treatment on me and brought up the matter of the children, asking when we were going to tell them. We decided to tell our girls the next day. I slept in and didn't go to church.

It was late morning when we gathered the girls together. I looked at them and said, "I don't know if you remember the lumps I had on my neck a while back?" They looked at each other and kind of nodded their heads. I continued, "Well, I had them taken out, you probably remember seeing the stitches after? Anyway, the doctor said I have some sort of sickness, that he is going to treat it, and I am going to be fine. I don't know what it will be like—we are going to stay right here and continue with our lives. I am going to be okay, and you are going to be okay." My wife sat there quietly and listened. Each of our daughters came over and gave me a hug and then went outside to play. At their young age, being sick meant having a cold or the flu, something I would recover from soon. I went to the grocery to get the ingredients for the caramelized ham steaks I was making that night. Over dinner, we continued normal conversation. My goal was to protect my children and not have them worry. As I fell into bed that night, I felt quite humbled by my lack of energy, something that I always had an abundance of through playing baseball and competing in wrestling much of my life. While I had always been a Christian, I don't recall ever praying for myself. My new reality was pushing me to think and act differently. I closed my eyes and said, "Lord, you know my situation, be there for me."

I woke up the next morning, on Monday, and returned to work. I still felt weak and tired, although the distraction of work helped me push through. As I started my second infusion, I was now feeling more vulnerable, more open to others around me. I started talking to the other patients sitting next to me, uncovering their stories and sharing mine. All of a sudden, the process felt purposeful. At one point in my life, I had wanted to become a minister. Listening to others and sharing how I felt during the chemotherapy treatments was a way to minister to others. In business, one of the reasons I am very successful is that I am very vulnerable. As I open up to others, they open up to me. This gave me strength and made me feel good inside, despite the toxic chemicals that were pumping through my veins. Each chemotherapy treatment yielded different people to sit with. As such, I did not develop any lasting relationships. When I was finished with my three-hour infusion,

I would feel nauseous and weak. Despite how I felt, I kept my philosophy of, "Don't ever give up" at the forefront of my mind. I had a family to support that was depending on me.

Early in my treatments, a close friend came over to visit. My friend is from California and a real wine connoisseur. We decided to go out to dinner at my favorite restaurant. I was far enough from the last infusion that I had some strength. We drank a bottle of wine with dinner and drank port wine with desert. It sounded like a really good idea at the time and for that evening, helped me imagine that I was healthy. By the time I got home, I was feeling nauseous, which turned into vomiting and diarrhea overnight. The next day, I received a letter in the mail from the hospital saying not to drink alcohol while on chemotherapy. How I wish I had known that when I started my treatment!

As each week progressed, I became more tired after the treatment. The good days of feeling like I had energy started to decrease in between my weekly chemotherapy infusions. Despite how I felt, I kept working, pushing myself through each day. I am a very competitive person and needed to be one of the top producers at work, whether I had cancer or not. Having distractions, like work, were super helpful and served a valuable purpose. As my hair started to fall out after week four, my vanity was rearing its head again—it was uncomfortable to see myself in the mirror, knowing that I now looked like a cancer patient.

My parents came to visit around this time. In an effort to try and protect them, I had not shared my news that I had cancer. My mother walked into the house and said, "What are you doing with your hair?"

I replied, "Oh, it's probably a different cut from the last time you saw me." As the weekend progressed, she noticed my lack of energy and knew that was very uncharacteristic of me. I finally decided it was best to tell them. The next morning, I said, "Mom and Dad, I have some news to share with you. I have been diagnosed with a low-grade lymphoma, and it is very treatable." My mom did just what I expected, started sobbing uncontrollably as she walked over to hug me. I actually didn't know at the time that my cancer was very treatable. It seemed important for all of us to have hope and imagine a positive outcome. And, thankfully, that is what turned out to be the case.

I continued having lunch with my seven male friends throughout my treatment, every Friday. I referred to them as my lunch group. We would show up every week and talk about what was going on. In 1979, cancer was a rare diagnosis and not something widely discussed. A guy in our group was going through a divorce during my treatment, and the focus was usually on him, rather than my cancer treatment. It felt like all the men were worried that if divorce could happen to him, maybe it could happen to them also. One day I decided to bring up my cancer and said, "Cancer is not contagious; you can't get it from me. It's okay for us to talk about it." Even though it was uncomfortable for them to talk about my cancer, I still looked forward to our lunches and felt supported by them. This group served an important purpose in my life.

Another group that I continued spending time with during my treatment was my men's group through the Pittsburg Experiment. The Pittsburgh Experiment (PX) is a nonprofit that convenes small groups of professionals in western Pennsylvania with the goal of connecting people and building positive relationships. I was able to share details with this group about my cancer experience, and they gave me tremendous support. They would pray for me and sometimes lay hands on me to lift me up. I didn't like being the focus of the group conversation, though. I preferred focusing on others in our group and praying for them, which strengthened my faith. This group supported me in so many ways and was pivotal to my ability to weather the storm called cancer.

Following my chemotherapy infusions, I had weekly radiation on my throat, neck, and the top of my chest for fifteen weeks. It made my voice extremely dry, and I had difficulty talking, likely due to the radiation burning my salivary glands. I carried around a bottle of water at all times during the day and took one to meetings with clients. Hearing my scratchy voice and seeing the bottle of water made for interesting conversations. In my effort to remain the vulnerable salesperson I had always been, I was honest with my clients about what I was enduring. They were stunned after hearing my story and amazed by my willingness to share. My voice finally came back after about six months.

My wife was a good mother and was supportive of me as I was going through treatment. As I gained enough strength, she encouraged me to start to exercise again. When I began to feel like myself again and the side effects had dissipated, my wife pulled away. She looked at me and said, "Your problems are too big for me. I know I am going to have my own problems in life, and I can't handle yours." I was shocked by her words and determined to keep our marriage together.

I tried everything I knew to save our marriage, but one day she said, "Stop. You don't understand. I don't love you anymore." As the words sunk in, it felt like a bucket of cement coming down on my head. I had just survived the worst—or what I thought was the worst—with the cancer treatment. It had never crossed my mind that our marriage would be a casualty of my cancer diagnosis.

As a strong Christian, I believe that God leads us on the path we are meant to go. I have always been a survivor, despite challenges, probably because of my strong faith. Within four years of my diagnosis, my wife asked for a divorce. It was important for me to let her stay in our home with the girls. A couple from the Pittsburg Experiment offered space in their home for me to live with them. I felt so supported by the ability to live in their home rather than renting an apartment by myself. They were loving and helpful to me in countless ways. My daughters and I even celebrated Thanksgiving with them. My daughters would stay with me one or two nights during the week and every weekend. Despite our irreconcilable differences, my wife and I ended up co-parenting in a collaborative way, including taking the girls to concerts together. It was important to me to put our differences aside and show a loving face to our girls, even though my wife thought that I had taken the best years of her life from her with my cancer treatment.

My journey since my first chemotherapy has not been without ups and downs. My cancer has come back four times. Since completing my first chemotherapy treatment, I have had a PET scan every six months. When I first started dating my second wife, I decided it was important for her to know about my history, given the experience I went through with my first wife. On our second date, I looked at her over dinner and said, "Before we get too involved, there is something I need to tell you."

She smiled and said, "Is it about your cancer?"

I was stunned by her response and said, "How did you know?"

She reached out, put her hand on mine, and said, "Oh, I heard about it through friends. Your cancer doesn't have anything to do with us and how I feel about you." I innately felt like I could trust and believe her; she was so humble and kind. In 1985, two years after I started dating her and while I was in remission, I was guided by God to a recurrence of the cancer, this time in my stomach. My doctor used the same treatment, R-Chop chemotherapy and radiation. While I endured my treatment, my girlfriend was always by my side, in a supportive and loving way. I was again in remission until 1991, when I felt lumps under my arm. My doctor used the same treatment once again. I survived and decided to marry my girlfriend in 1992. I was in remission until 1998, when I noticed something wasn't right with my groin. This time, my doctor chose a different treatment, called Rituxan. I cherished the moments and days in between the recurrences and found strength each time to endure more treatment. I was very active in my community, willing to share my story with anyone who would listen. I was asked to join the board of directors of the Leukemia and Lymphoma Society, where I was afforded opportunities to witness to many patients and families. I was then voted president of the Western Pennsylvania and Northern West Virginia chapter. I was again in remission until 2005, when the radiologist saw nodes in my abdomen area on my PET scan. My doctor chose the Rituxan treatment again.

I have been in remission now for fourteen years, despite one scare in 2015. My doctor continues to introduce me as "the longest living survivor with non-Hodgkin's lymphoma." That feels like quite a weight to bear, although I am up for the challenge. After all, there is a reason God saved me—to nurture others and give them hope through sharing my story.

I am often asked when I speak to patients going through treatment or to large audiences, "How are you getting through?"

My answer is always the same. "I am a very optimistic person, and I believe that I am going to get through anything just fine. I have a strong faith that guides me every day." When I was going through treatment the first time in 1979, I prayed to God that he let me live until my children graduated from high school. When my last daughter graduated, I prayed again, saying "God, I think I misspoke. I need to reevaluate my request, because I meant to say graduate from college." Before I knew it, I was watching my youngest daughter graduate from college.

Between my wife and me, we have thirteen grandchildren. I feel like I am thriving, in part because of my wife, and despite the setbacks and reentering treatment along the way. Life is a complicated journey that sometimes unfolds in unimaginable ways. If we surrender and embrace it, taking one day at a time, it can be rewarding and fulfilling. I now know how important it is to be prepared in all aspects of life, including the trials and tribulations. I believe God still has more work for me to do; my part is putting one foot in front of the other each day and moving forward. Sitting on the other side of the treatment, I am able to fully grasp the reality that, until I personally experienced it, I would not have ever fully comprehended its physical impacts. It touched every part of my being—mind, body, and spirit. There were the visible side effects and the silent ones, like the gut-wrenching nausea.

Four years ago, in 2015, the PET scan showed I had cancer in my breast. "But wait, doctor, I am a man. How could that be?" They told me it was a definite diagnosis, not a mistake. I endured several mammograms and the technician had to squeeze really hard to get a good image of my breast. The mammograms showed a cancerous tumor in my nipple. I was in disbelief, and all of a sudden felt extreme empathy for women who have to endure these very uncomfortable mammograms. My doctor scheduled surgery, given my previous history. For some reason, the doctor called one day before the surgery and asked me to come back to the hospital for another mammogram and a biopsy. Following the tests, the radiologist asked to meet with me. He sat me down and showed me the images. He was stunned, staring at the image and back at me. He turned to me and said, "Bill, you must have healed your body. There is no sign of the cancer." He recommended I go through genetic testing, which I did. The results came back negative. I am still perplexed by how or why this experience happened, although I am grateful that the end result was no surgery or treatment.

Also in 2015, I learned that one of my Friday lunch group friends was dying of cancer. I went to see him with a couple of our other lunch group friends to say our good-byes. Once I was alone with him, I asked if he would be okay if I prayed with him. He smiled and said, "Bill, I would really appreciate that. What a nice thing to offer." I reached out and held his hand, then started praying. Being able to pray with him was one of the most meaningful experiences I have had. It felt like it made a difference to him as well.

In 2017, I was having trouble walking straight and was experiencing thinking and reasoning problems. My doctor didn't think it was the lymphoma, so he ordered some tests. I learned that my spinal fluid was not doing what it was supposed to do. Several times I had to go in for a test where they withdrew forty ccs of spinal fluid and then had me walk across the room. I was finally diagnosed with normal pressure hydrocephalus, which typically occurs in individuals in their mid-eighties. After enduring several recurrences with cancer, my tolerance and acceptance for health issues had increased. I had a shunt surgically implanted in my brain that serves to normalize the spinal fluid. The downside is the sciatic pain down my leg, although I am grateful to have a physical therapist who comes to my house to work with me weekly. I recently had a spinal cord stimulator put in my back. *Here is one more health-related challenge, forcing me to surrender and let go.* I feel as if God is trying to teach me humility, upping the ante on what I am capable of overcoming. As a result, my prayer days have become stronger and stronger, praying at a deeper level and several times a day, including first thing in the morning and just before bed. I am convinced that I am still here because of my faith, my willingness to accept my path, and my positive attitude.

Advice for Others

How I supported myself
- Kept working, which was a helpful distraction.
- Prayed every day.
- Stayed involved in the church, kept serving in my roles.
- Kept mowing grass until we moved, then outsourced the mowing.
- Got together and prayed with friends.

How others supported me
- My current wife, family, and daughters were extremely supportive and loving, always there.
- My manager and other coworkers were very supportive.
- The Pittsburg Experiment men's group would pray for me and gave me tremendous support; then I would focus on others and pray for them, which helped me spiritually.
- A couple from the Pittsburg Experiment made space in their home for me to live when I went through my divorce.

- I met with my lunch group weekly, and while we didn't talk about the cancer, I felt supported by them, and the weekly ritual served a purpose in my life.

Helpful tips
- If you are a partner or a spouse of someone who learns of a diagnosis, think about the questions you have and the right time and place to ask them; in front of the patient is not always the best choice.
- Be aware that if you have been diagnosed, family members and friends sometimes put distance between you and shy away, as if the cancer is contagious.
- While I only got one opinion clinically, I highly recommend getting a second opinion, whether if it is surgery or a cancer diagnosis.
- If you or a loved one is facing a cancer diagnosis, ask what you are able to keep doing, such as eating, and what you need to stop doing, like drinking.

VALERIE'S STORY

———— • ● • ————

It was the early evening of a snowy day on January 15, 2012, and we had already eaten dinner. I was taking a bubble bath with my six-year-old daughter in my claw foot bathtub, something we did often. The tub was oversized, similar to a deep well with extra tall sides. With my family history of my mom having had breast cancer, I was scheduled to start having mammograms at age forty and had one scheduled for the end of the month. My doctor thought it was important, and honestly, I had not been very diligent about doing my monthly self-exams. On this particular evening, my daughter had a couple of Barbies with her in the tub and was playing around, holding each one on the top edge of the tub and then plunging them into the bubbles. As the first Barbie went into the water, I lay back and looked down at the water. As I did, I could see something protruding from my breast. It was a perfectly round, green-pea-sized lump that looked kind of like a swollen bug bite with raised skin. My daughter was squealing with joy, lost in her play and intently focused on her diving Barbies; she didn't notice what I was doing. I looked at her and looked back down at this new discovery. Different thoughts started racing through my mind: *Oh, it's nothing . . . It couldn't be cancer, it's too small . . . It couldn't be cancer because it hurts to the touch.* My head felt like it was spinning out of control as thought after thought raced through my mind for what felt like a half hour, although it was probably only five minutes.

A big splash brought my focus back to the tub. It was time for my daughter to go to bed, so we stepped out onto the bath-mat, toweled off, and got into our pajamas. My daughter was in a phase where she preferred Mommy to put her to bed. We walked down the hall into her room for our normal bedtime routine after a bath—read a book and then say prayers. We always said prayers together. While thoughts raced through my mind—*This can't be, I'm too young*—I kept a calm face to my daughter as if it were a normal bedtime. When we finished and she had closed her eyes, I turned on the sound machine next to her bed, kissed her forehead, and clicked on the night light. I gingerly walked out of her room and down the hall to my room. My husband was sitting on the bed watching TV. I asked him to come in the bathroom to look at what I had discovered. He quickly jumped up, came in, and looked at the raised bump. He said, in a somewhat concerned voice, "Honey, I think you should go and get it checked out, just to be sure." He wrapped his arms around me as we both processed what this could mean. We had grown much closer after surviving deep losses over the past several years with the deaths of our two children. Thoughts of what this lump could be started flooding my mind as I fell into bed: *No way could a tumor be that small, could it be? Mom's tumor was the size of a golf ball.* I closed my eyes and started talking to God and praying, "God, we have survived so much loss. This just can't be happening again. Please make it be okay and give me the strength to get through this." I had a fitful sleep as I tossed and turned most of the night.

The next morning, I took our children over to my friend's house for a play date. I got them settled and made sure they were engrossed in a game, and then went into the kitchen where my friend was standing. I walked over to her and said quietly, "Would you feel this?" I pointed to the lump on my breast. I had nursed my daughter until she was three years old and thought maybe it was just a clogged duct. She felt it and said, "Oh yes, Valerie, that is something to get checked out. Why don't you call your doctor right now and make an appointment?" I trusted her advice and pulled out my phone. As I dialed the number I thought, *I have no time for this, no time for cancer.* Because I had lost two children, my doctor always worked me in quickly. I scheduled an appointment for the day after next.

I did my best to keep busy until the appointment, although my fear kept trying to command my attention. A friend of mine offered to watch my children while I went to the appointment. Before I knew it, I was sitting in the doctor's office, waiting. When the doctor came into the exam room, I showed her the lump and asked her opinion. She did a full breast exam, and then said, "Yes, Valerie, that is really suspicious looking. I know you have a mammogram scheduled in two weeks. Let's not wait; I will get you scheduled for tomorrow." The next morning, I arrived for my mammogram. My husband had asked me if I wanted him to come, and I had said no. I found myself waiting for what seemed like a long time after the technician finished with my mammogram.

When you have a mammogram and they don't come back right away, there is usually something wrong. My heart started racing and the fear started welling in my mind: *Please, dear God, don't let this be true. I am so young. Oh my, I don't want to have to tell my parents. Are they going to be able to handle this?* I could feel my breathing getting short and knew I needed my husband. I called him and said, "Honey, you need to come over now. I need you." He stopped what he was doing and rushed to the hospital. I watched as each woman who had come in after me was being released as "good to go." I was still waiting and began to panic, pacing the floor, and staring at the door every time it opened. My husband arrived and was told to wait outside in the big waiting room. Finally, the nurse called me back and said that I needed an ultrasound.

I walked into the ultrasound room feeling a little dizzy. As the technician started the ultrasound, I felt as if I was outside of my body, observing but not feeling. He took several pictures and then asked me to wait while he talked to the doctor. A radiologist came in the room and sat down. After introducing himself, he said "I am concerned about this lump right here. When it is a cyst, it is solid black. When it is a tumor, there is blood flow. As you can see, it is not solid black. We are going to need a biopsy." I started to feel numb, thinking, *This can't be happening.* They were able to fit me into the schedule and do the biopsy about an hour later. I went out to the waiting room to sit with my husband. We held hands and tried to distract ourselves with watching TV. I called my friend and asked if she could watch the kids longer, as it might take several more hours. The nurse called me back pretty quickly. I took a deep breath and lay down on the table. It was a pretty straightforward biopsy since the tumor was so small and it went by fast. I was still feeling dizzy and now getting nauseous as I dressed to go home.

As I drove home, thoughts started racing through my mind again: *I am really in disbelief that this is happening to me, I'm too young. Between losing my babies and my daughter being born and my husband having his two hip surgeries, I am completely drained emotionally. There is no way this can be happening.* I was confused and completely baffled as I reflected on the unfolding of the events of the past few days. When I got home and my husband walked in after me, I said anxiously, "People just don't have this many things happen in their life. If this is cancer, how are we going to tell our parents?"

He wrapped his arms around me, which felt calming and comforting, just what I needed. He looked at me and said, "Honey, we are not going to think about what could be right now and how we will tell our parents. There is no sense in alarming anyone yet." I was so grateful that he was being the voice of reason. I kept asking him "What if?" questions, and he kept saying we were going to take it one step at a time.

Anxiety pulsed through my veins that night as I recounted what our family had endured over the past five years. In addition to my husband's two surgeries, I had been pregnant twice before my youngest daughter was born. With one, a daughter, I experienced a difficult pregnancy and went into shock twice and almost died. I was induced at twenty-six weeks, and due to several conditions, my daughter died shortly thereafter. Two years later, I then became pregnant with a boy and had a joyful, easy pregnancy. I was really looking forward to welcoming him into our lives, until he was stillborn at thirty-eight weeks, on October 17. My body was producing a lot of milk, and I would pump every day. I was struggling to make it through each hour, feeling such deep grief, and needed to find some purpose in all the loss I was experiencing. One night, God spoke to me and guided me to donate the milk to triplets in Minnesota. Focusing on pumping and donating the milk gave me a purpose. It really helped me heal.

The next morning, I looked at my husband and said, "We have a beautiful baby boy. I am never going to try and have a baby again." I was using birth control at the time. I learned very quickly that God's plan was different. A few months later, I started to feel nauseous and was hungry all the time. I thought it was just from pumping milk. And when it didn't go away, I went to the doctor.

I was shocked to learn I was pregnant. It was the last thing on my mind. I called my husband in tears, and he said, "This is the best news ever!" His words permeated my heart, and I knew he was right. We embraced our new reality, unsure of what all this loss and now a new beginning meant for us. We welcomed our baby girl Bailey eight months later and celebrated our new reality.

My doctor's office called three days after the biopsy to say the results had come back inconclusive, despite having two different labs examine the tissue sample. She recommended sending the sample to Tennessee to have another pathology group evaluate the sample, which sounded like a good next step. I did my best to keep busy with my children, work, and the house, although my mind would wander sometimes to "What if?" When it did, I would call my husband, and he would calm me down.

A week later, I was at preschool teaching, reading to my class. I was engrossed in the story and discussion until I noticed someone standing near our reading circle. I looked up and saw my director, who motioned to me that I had a phone call. I walked my children over to the class next door and asked the teacher to watch them; then I went downstairs to the office. I picked up the phone and heard my doctor's voice on the other end. She had just received the test results back from Tennessee. I took a deep breath. Then she said, "I am sorry to say that I have bad news. It turns out that you do have cancer, and it is fast growing. The reason the other tests were inconclusive is because you have a cancerous tumor encased inside noncancerous skin. I need to refer you to an oncologist and recommend you go see him quickly." As I stood there listening to these words, tears started streaming from my eyes. Just when I thought things couldn't get worse, they did.

Cheryl, the director of my preschool, looked over at me and could see my tears. She went up to get my purse so the children wouldn't see me crying. She brought it to me, looked at me with compassion in her eyes, and said, "Valerie, I can see that something is going on that you need to focus on. You go and do whatever you need to do. I will finish out your class."

I went out the back door, and once I was in my car, I dialed my husband's number as my hands were shaking. I shared the news with him between sobs. I still remember that moment like it was yesterday. He was pretty quiet and didn't say very much, although I could hear the devastation in his voice. I looked at my watch and noticed the time, then told my husband that I would pick up our son and daughter and see him at home later. Neither of us had many words in this moment. When I arrived home, I dialed my parents' phone number. My mother said, "Hi, honey, what's up?"

In an effort to keep my conversation light and upbeat, I said, "Hi, Mom. Oh, that's right, Dad is still at work. When he gets home, will you both give me a call? I look forward to talking with you. I love you." We had a joke in our family about how my aunt and uncle would always get on the phone together whenever I called them, no matter what I called about. That had given me an idea. I did not want to tell one parent before the other.

A couple of hours later, my phone rang. Both of my parents were on the phone. I said, "I have some news to share with you. I have just been diagnosed with breast cancer. We caught it very early, although it is fast growing."

There was silence from my father. Then my mother said, "You know what, honey? It's all going to be okay."

My father was more emotional. All he said was, "I can't believe this is happening," and he got off the phone. He told me later that he cried for hours. When there were no more tears, he turned on his computer and started looking for plane tickets to come visit. He had a part-time job that he could get covered, and my mom was retired. He called me back and said, "We are coming to be with you and will stay as long as you need us. I love you."

The burden of my diagnosis and what my parents must have been going through left me an emotional wreck. I was absorbed in the moment, between talking to them and still sorting out the news in my mind. Then I happened to glance at my watch and realized it was time to pick up my children. My son was eleven, which was old enough to know something was wrong. He is pretty aware of his surroundings and able to pick up emotions from others. I knew he would be able to see the sadness on my face, so I did my best to smile as we walked through his school to the car. I buckled my daughter in her car seat and helped my son get buckled, and then I drove toward home. As I drove, we talked about their day and what had happened at school. Then I said, "I have some news to share with you both. I have just been diagnosed with cancer. The good news is Big (grandad) and Gammy (grandma) are coming to stay for a while!" My son was very quiet all the way home, as if he was sorting out the words he had heard me say. My daughter likely didn't know what having cancer meant and went back to playing with her toy. A hush fell over the inside of our car as I drove.

When we were home and in the house, my son looked at me and asked, "Does this mean you're going to die?" *Wow, there it was out in the open, the word* die, I thought. I was not prepared for that question and found it really hard to look at my son. I felt a stabbing feeling in my gut. I wanted so to protect both my children, shield them from pain, and my son especially, as he had endured all of the previous losses with us. I dug deep for strength and said, "The doctors are going to do the very best to get this out of me and give me medicine to heal." I wrapped my arms around him as we both cried. Soon after, my husband walked in the door from work. He came over and wrapped his arms around us as tears streamed down our cheeks. Despite the news of the day, we quickly got busy with cooking dinner and helping our son with homework. My son took the news really hard at first, and my daughter seemed to be doing okay, although at six years old, I am not sure she understood what being diagnosed with cancer meant.

My doctor's office made an appointment for me with the oncologist within a couple of days. As my husband and I were waiting, he started telling jokes and making me laugh, which lightened my mood and distracted me from where we were. The nurse called us back, and as I walked to the exam room, I felt a small sense of comfort, knowing that we were about to learn more and be able to move forward soon. The doctor introduced himself and explained, "Valerie, your tumor is fast growing and aggressive. The good news is we caught it so early, and it is so small. That means a good prognosis is likely possible." I took a big deep breath, feeling relieved to know a little more. He continued, "You will need a lumpectomy."

Okay, so that sounds better than a mastectomy, I thought. "Will I need to have chemotherapy and radiation?" I asked.

He gave me a compassionate look, wanting to offer hope, although also wanting to be transparent. "I really don't know yet. Let's start with the surgeon and lumpectomy and see what we learn." I felt the muscles in my neck start to relax slightly, hearing I might not have to endure chemotherapy and radiation. He said his office would schedule the lumpectomy as soon as possible, and he would be in touch. As we left, my sense of calm quickly dissipated as my mind raced forward two steps to, *What if I don't survive?* My life had changed forever, and the path forward was still unknown.

I was able to meet with the surgeon two days later, which was helpful. Progressing through the steps quickly enabled me to quiet my mind and stay focused on the present. The surgeon explained what was involved in the procedure: she would try to get a certain amount of tissue and also test my lymph nodes for any signs of the cancer spreading. While I was grateful to learn more and feel a little in control, my spirit was deflated when I heard the procedure would not happen until the following week. *Really? Why can't they just cut it out today? Waiting will make me go crazy*, I thought. Each day seemed to last longer, and the uneasy feeling in my stomach became more extreme, causing me to lose my appetite. I kept as busy as I could to distract myself, although I imagine I was an edgy and unpleasant person to be around during that week. The bright part of my week was welcoming my parents to our home. I felt comforted and supported having them close, especially with all the loss we had already endured.

Treatment Experience

I arrived at the hospital for the lumpectomy, and all went as planned, including the surgeon taking samples from two of my lymph nodes. The surgeon said she would send the tissue samples to a pathology group in California, and it would take several days to process. When I was getting dressed to go home, the surgeon explained that she was going to put my arm in a sling in order to help the incision site heal quickly. She recommended I go home and take it easy, meaning I was not supposed to wash dishes or do loads of laundry, mostly rest. I thanked her and we headed home, feeling a small sense of relief that another step in the process was complete. When I walked into my house, my mind started racing again. *What if we get bad news? What if I am really facing chemother-apy and radiation, how will that impact our family, our lives?* For my friends who know me, I am not comfortable just resting. I feel like I am being lazy, like I am failing at my job as a mother and a wife. Keeping busy and doing chores around the house helped distract me and helped me feel like I was in control, as I waited for results I had no control over.

The next night, as I waited on the test results, my crazy mind started to spin out of control. I woke up feeling dizzy and discon-nected, like I needed to get up and do something. I quietly climbed out of bed and tiptoed out of my room and into the kitchen. I opened the pantry, grabbed the broom and started sweeping at eleven at night. With two young children, I was usually asleep from exhaustion by then. As I swept the floor, I focused intently on sweeping every speck of dirt off the floor, as that was the only thing I felt in control of in that moment. When I felt like the floor was clean, I put the broom up and quietly crawled back into bed.

As I was pulling on my shirt over my head the next morning, I happened to glance down and notice that my incision site looked different, a little elevated from the day before. *Oh it is probably nothing, just a little swollen from the procedure and just now showing up. Probably nothing to worry about,* I thought. I quickly became immersed in the activities of the day with teaching preschool and caring for my children. After dinner, I felt something odd in my chest, as if there was something wet pooling under my shirt. I stepped into the bathroom and turned on the light to check it out. I looked down and saw gushing brown blood from my chest through my shirt. I started screaming, "Dad, I need help. Come quick!" I was so grateful my dad was around since he is comfortable dealing with blood, and the sight of blood makes my husband squeamish. As I started hyperventilating over what this might mean, that my treatment start date may get delayed, my dad calmed me down and called the doctor. The on-call doctor recommended that I tape up the incision site with butterfly tape from the first aid kit and come in the next day to get it checked out. Here I was, being a noncompliant patient, overdoing it physically and not sitting around as the surgeon had instructed me to. I thanked my dad and went up to bed. As I lay down, I closed my eyes and prayed, "God, please help my body heal quickly so I am able to start treatment on time. Forgive me for not listening to my orders." I continued to pray morning, noon, and at night before bed, wanting a miracle that I could start radiation quickly, if I needed it.

The next morning, the doctor's office called and asked me to come in the office to discuss the treatment plan. My husband and I showed up for the appointment and were called right back. My doctor pulled up the results and said, "Valerie, the results show that you have intraductal carcinoma. It is a fast and aggressive type of cancer. The good news is there is no sign of cancer in your lymph nodes, which means it has not spread." He took a deep breath and continued, "You actually have a choice in terms of treatment. Your results are on the cusp of needing radiation and chemotherapy, meaning you could choose to go through it or not. We have options to consider, and I think it's important to do all that we can to make this go away." As I sat there sorting out everything my doctor had just shared, I closed my eyes and said a prayer, wanting guidance from God on what our next step should be. I looked at the doctor and said, "So what kind of chemotherapy would you recommend and how long will I be in treatment?" My doctor explained the options and we developed a plan, which included radiation and chemotherapy. I wanted to do all I could to increase my chances of survival. He said he could get me in a clinical trial for radiation, which would be twice a day for five days. While that seemed intense, it felt better to me emotionally to only have one week of radiation, rather than feeling like it was going on forever.

As my husband drove us home from the appointment, I started to reflect on how this situation had happened that I developed cancer. I remembered back to the day that my mother and I went in for genetic counseling and testing, thinking the results would be the definitive answer. While we both tested negative for a genetic link to cancer, we each developed cancer nonetheless. It was a great reminder to us both that genetic testing is just one piece of the overall puzzle of risk factors for cancer. A few hours later, I heard from my doctor that I would be able to participate in the radiation clinical trial. I was able to start it in a couple of weeks.

While I was happy to have the radiation all in one week, I'd underestimated how grueling and taxing on my body it would be. I developed nausea immediately and was extremely tired. My dad would take me to the morning appointment, I would come home and sleep before the afternoon appointment; then I would go to sleep when I came home after the second appointment. Every day I would wake up feeling depleted as I faced the next set of treatments. The five days seemed to last forever. When I reached the end of the week, I felt many psychological benefits of having the radiation happen all in one week—it limited my feeling of being sick since it was over so quickly, and it helped my mind shift to positivity.

I had heard that when you start on chemotherapy treatment, you will find a clump of hair on your pillow on day fourteen. I had my first infusion of Taxol chemotherapy, and sure enough, I awoke on day fourteen looking at hair on my pillow. I was grateful to have had that warning and knew what I had planned to do. When I picked up my son and daughter from school, I took them wig shopping. They wanted to be with me, and I appreciated not being alone. When I brought my wig home, the next step was shaving my head. My son did not want any part of this process, but my six-year-old daughter did, so she joined me in my bathroom. My hair was a little below my shoulders at the time. I looked in the mirror, taking in the picture I showed to the world, knowing it would be forever changed. I said a prayer for strength and first started by cutting my hair really short. My daughter watched with huge eyes as pieces of my hair fell to the ground. She walked over and picked up some strands, holding them in her hands. Next I picked up the razor. Although tears were welling up in my eyes, I knew I wanted to show a strong face to my daughter, so I held them back. Having her in the room with me felt so supportive. I looked in the mirror again when my head was shaved, taking in my baldness as the reality of my new look permeated my soul. Then the mom in me looked at the reflection of my daughter, sitting there staring while she held strands of my hair. It was such a surreal moment, and one I will never forget.

My son was quiet when he saw me with my bald head after I was finished. I decided to change the subject and focus our attention on his helping me cook dinner to lighten our mood. I chose to wear a wig during the school year for appearances, but during the summer months, I was comfortable with my bald head. Seeing me without hair was a little awkward for my son. I could tell by how he wouldn't look at my face when I wasn't wearing my wig. When I went to the grocery store, I would notice people staring at me, and when I looked back at them, they would tilt their lips up slightly, kind of half grins. I felt strong and empowered, but others were awkward around me.

As I finished chemotherapy, I reflected on how well cared for I felt, once I let others in to support me. I was overwhelmed by the outpouring of love and compassion I experienced. I surrounded myself with people who love me unconditionally. Six of my friends, who have been together since my son was little, would work with each other and figure out a plan to show up at my house, always just when I needed support. We would lie on the bed together, and they would hold my hand or rub my feet with lotion. I always felt relaxed when they came over, as I knew I didn't have to entertain them. We were raising our children together, experiencing life together. I felt immensely thankful for the grace of so much help. Feeling their love and support so deeply in my heart really kept me strong.

In addition to my husband, my parents and my mother-in-law were my rock and inspiration to keep going every day. My parents came to live with me once I was diagnosed, wanting to be at my side through everything. My dad was able to stay for three months and went to every appointment with me so my husband could focus on work. My mom's visit was cut short when her mother fell and needed help. My mom was one of my biggest supporters during my treatment, both as a breast cancer survivor and as someone who exuded positivity; she really helped me get through each day, one step at a time. When my mom had to leave, my mother-in-law came to town to help. My dad took care of me, driving me to appointments and helping me in between and afterward. My mother-in-law took care of driving my children to school and activities and helped them after school while my husband worked. When I reflect on this experience, I can now see the positive impact of having my parents and mother-in-law close as we all lived through this challenge. This experience permeated every part of our lives—there was not a stone unturned, not a connection left hanging. Watching their mom, their rock of Gibraltar, not look like their mom anymore helped my children gain deep life perspective at a much younger age than most. Living through this experience as a family created a new normal for us, a different perspective on what is and what life means.

The cancer treatment process strengthened my faith to depths unimaginable to me before. I am now much more vigilant about spending time in my own Bible study, reading scripture each morning. It is now my first ritual of the day and is protected as sacred. Nothing else gets in the way. After all we had been through as a family, it felt like my most available option was to surrender to God and allow Him to lead me through this process. I was grateful to be able to take a leave of absence from work and focus on my healing, which made a big difference. This experience reminded me how important community is, as we were blessed with countless acts of kindness and support. Our community stepped in to help with our kids and house chores. For me personally, having three months with my dad, side by side through each step, was one of the greatest blessings from the experience, one I will cherish in my heart forever. Our nuclear family—my husband, two children, and I—would sometimes cling to each other through the toughest moments, deepening our bond and love for each other. We lived through periods of time where friends and neighbors stepped in to run the household, such as cooking and doing the laundry when I was at my worst and suffering debilitating side effects. I am one of those people who believes that I have to do everything myself without asking for anything. Once we shared the news of my diagnosis with friends, I had many people reach out and offer to help with food or running errands. I graciously declined at first, as the voice inside me said I was a bad mother, a bad wife if I was not the one doing everything. I said no several times and finally prayed to be able to surrender. It was really hard for me to give in, to let go and let others help. Once I did, my friends willingly stepped in and took over my life, giving me peace and space to heal.

Advice for Others

How I supported myself
- Prayed several times a day.
- Started each day with Bible studies and reading at home.
- Spent as much time with my close friends and family as I could.
- On days when I felt strong, I spent time outside.
- I worked in my flower bed when I could.

How others supported me
- I had a strong, supportive husband who was always there for me.
- My parents came to live with me to support and comfort me.
- My sister came to visit when she could, and I felt supported by her.
- My six close friends figured out a schedule to come by and see me; I didn't have to entertain them; we would lie on the bed or they would rub my feet.

- One friend organized a meal train, and families from the preschool also organized meals.

Helpful tips
- When you see someone who has a look about them that something is out of place, tell them they look great, that they have a great smile or something like that; don't be afraid to speak up and break the silence.
- When someone wants to help you, let them come into your life and do whatever they want to help you, be open and willing to surrender, regardless of the situation.

DAN'S STORY

———— • ● • ————

I had been having regular colonoscopies since I was twenty years old as part of the ongoing evaluation of my colitis. My gastroenterologist had informed me that there was an increased risk of colon cancer due to my disease, although they did not think it was something I needed to think about in my twenties and thirties. As I approached my mid-forties, my colitis was well under control, and all of a sudden, I had let eight years go by without a checkup, right as I was approaching the magic age of fifty. Colorectal cancer is the second leading cause of death from cancer in the United States, with an estimated 50,000 deaths each year. While the incidence of disease is increasing in younger populations, the vast majority of individuals with a new diagnosis are forty-five and older. The American Cancer Society recommends that individuals with average risk of colon cancer start being screened at age forty-five, given no other symptoms. There are now several options for how to be screened.

My real reason—actually my excuse—for not getting screened for colon cancer was that I felt too busy to make time. There were just too many things going on in my life to take a day off for a simple colonoscopy that could have caught my cancer earlier, perhaps even in the pre-cancerous stage. At age forty-five, I had major heart surgery to repair a defective mitral valve. This involved taking my heart out of my body, cutting it open, and then manually repairing the valve. A year later, I changed jobs, which required relocation from Colorado to Nashville. We had to sell our beautiful home and find a new place to live in a city where we didn't know anyone. My wife and I both commuted back and forth on weekends until she was able to get a transfer. And we also decided to build a new house in Nashville, which ended up taking two years to complete.

So other health issues, selling our house, moving to a new state, building a new home, and the challenge of a new job kept me focused elsewhere and operating in a high-stress mode. But it really wasn't that I was too busy, it was that other priorities dominated my life, causing me to put an important cancer screening on the back burner.

Luckily though, a couple of angels tapped me on my shoulder ironically at two different music events, which prompted me to get a colonoscopy probably just in time. The first angel came in the form of our next-door neighbor, Jamie O'Neal. Jamie is a famous singer-songwriter and member of the Grand Ole Opry, one of whose many hits happens to be "When I Think about Angels." One night in 2008, my wife and I went to see her perform. About halfway through her performance, Jamie introduced one of her band members, Charlie Kelly. Charlie approached the microphone and announced that he had recently been diagnosed with colon cancer. He also shared that his wife, Nan Kelly, host of CMA television, was also in the audience and she too was fighting cancer. I remember thinking how hard it must be for a husband and wife to have cancer at the same time. Charlie then went on to talk about his colon cancer diagnosis and treatment. Then he performed a song called "I Am Less of an Ass," a tongue-in-cheek piece he had written since his treatment, which included surgery to remove a part of his colon. As he sang the song, all of a sudden, I realized that it had been many years since my last colonoscopy. A few seconds later, my wife nudged me and whispered, "When did you have your last colonoscopy?" I whispered that I couldn't remember and immediately added it to my to-do list in my phone.

Despite making the note to schedule the colonoscopy, another two weeks went by and I still had not taken action. My wife and I continued with our busy lives, including a date night to go listen to live music at the famous Bluebird Cafe. We arrived and saw another couple already sitting at our four-top table, people we didn't know. It was common practice when attending a show at the Bluebird Café to be seated with others if your party is less than the number your table holds. Before we could even start small talk, the woman stared at me and asked, "How old are you? When was the last time you had a colonoscopy?"

I was quite startled with her direct question but quickly pulled out my mobile phone and gestured to it. "It's been too long. See I have it listed right here on my to-do list." I continued, "I am quite curious, why did you ask me?"

She gave me a very determined look and replied, "My first husband died of colon cancer, and I am on a mission to make sure as many people get screened as possible so that they have a different outcome." As the words she said settled into my mind, I started to wonder, *Is this divine intervention? Two times in two weeks, the topic of colon cancer has come up with total strangers.* I knew it was time to make an appointment and called the gastroenterologist she recommended the next day.

The morning of the procedure, my wife dropped me off and said she would see me in an hour or two. As the anesthesia permeated my veins, I quickly dozed off. The doctor started the procedure but quickly stopped about five minutes in when he found a large tumor a short distance from the lower part of the colon, in the colorectal area. The staff began calling my wife, but it took a number of attempts to reach her since her phone's ringer was turned off. She had been expecting the procedure to last at least an hour and a half before she was to return.

Still groggy from the anesthesia, I joined my wife in the doctor's office. He looked at me and in a compassionate voice said, "Dan, the reason I stopped the procedure so quickly was I found a very large mass in your colon." He went on to explain that they had taken a biopsy and would send it to the lab for testing. He then said he thought there was a 99 percent chance that the mass was cancer, and by the size of it, he believed it had been there quite some time. He also said that the chances of it having spread were high. All of a sudden, I was pinching myself wondering if I was dreaming and still in the procedure under the fog of the anesthesia. As the words sank in, thoughts started racing through my mind: *Oh my God, seriously, I am only fifty-two. Did he just say I have cancer?* My focus returned to the room, and I noticed he was not looking at me; instead he was directing all of his conversation to my wife, which increased my fears that I had terminal cancer.

We both left the office in shock. As my wife drove me home, the word "cancer" continued to permeate both of our minds as silence filled the air. *It is most likely cancer,* I thought. *What is my prognosis and how long do I have to live?* From a place of disbelief, I quickly shifted to anger, and then fear began to spread to every cell in my body. The muscles in my shoulders tensed up even more, and my stomach was turning over like clothes in a dryer. As we arrived home, a feeling of numbness overcame me. I was stunned. I had no answers and no control over my situation in that moment, which was a very hopeless feeling. My thoughts shifted to thinking about my wife and how to help her deal with the news—and the future. I began trying to comfort her and talk through important things like life insurance and selling the house. I am sure I wasn't making much sense, jumping ahead, given the lack of knowledge of what the future held for us. I'm not sure how or if I slept that night. The next morning, the doctor's office called to say they had put a rush on the pathology results and wanted me to come back the next day to meet with the doctor. While I was feeling grateful for the quick turnaround, waiting even for one day felt like life was moving in slow motion. As my mind would start to race forward, I would take a deep breath. I would start to focus on a work project or read an email, only to forget where I was, not knowing how much time had passed.

My wife and I went in the next morning to meet with the doctor. In a compassionate tone, he said, "Dan, the results have come back as I had thought—you have colorectal cancer." He continued to explain that he wouldn't know the stage until he conducted further tests. He referred me to an oncologist and also said that in all likelihood I would need surgery. He recommended a surgeon for a consultation and informed me that he was one of the best in town. He turned his focus to his phone, dialed a number, and reached the surgeon's office, only to learn that he was booked for over nine months out. He asked to speak directly with the surgeon. After a few minutes, the surgeon was on the phone. Following my doctor's explanation of my case and the urgency of my situation, the surgeon agreed to see me the following week.

A couple of short weeks before, I had learned that my position at work had been eliminated in a restructuring effort. I had a second interview over lunch set up immediately following my doctor's visit that day. As I sat in my car outside the restaurant, I worried about my ability to get through the conversation without breaking down. I took a few deep breaths and then I thought of my new reality and my wife, knowing I needed to stay strong. In view of my diagnosis, I was determined to keep a job with health insurance. Somehow, I was able to compartmentalize my health situation and stay positive and focused during the interview. I was delighted to receive a formal job offer the next day. As my thoughts raced forward to this new job, I was able to breathe a sigh of relief and relax a little, knowing my job with health insurance would continue.

The next week, my wife and I met with the surgeon. I was comforted by his calm demeanor when he came into the exam room. He introduced himself with a compassionate approach, and then explained the type of surgery I needed in great detail. When he was finished, he sat down and said, "I am not going anywhere until I answer all of your questions." We continued the dialogue for a while, and my wife and I were able to ask our many questions. When we had our questions answered, he stood up and said, "I want to show you what you are dealing with here." He picked up the flexible sigmoidoscope, had me lie down, and started a procedure. And there it was on the screen, the baseball-sized tumor. All of a sudden, I felt like I was in a documentary. I was looking at this tumor, knowing it was the enemy. I was squirming on the table as the reality set in that this was my body we were looking at. He finished the consult by explaining that before he performed the surgery, he recommended I undergo radiation and chemotherapy to shrink the tumor as much as possible, in hopes of getting "clear margins." As we said good-bye, the muscles in my neck relaxed slightly, for I felt confident that I had a compassionate and very qualified surgeon that I could trust.

Next, we met with the oncologist who explained the details of my test results and the treatment plan. She said I had stage II colon cancer, as the tumor had pierced the colon wall. I was to start with the Folfox drug regiment, which was a combination of drugs, and would receive the chemotherapy continually through a fanny pack and port for sixteen weeks. I was then to start radiation treatments twice a week halfway through receiving the chemotherapy. Post-surgery, her recommendation was to receive chemotherapy infusions every three weeks for six months.

Treatment Experience

The first step in my treatment plan was to have a port-a-cath surgically implanted in my chest that would allow a tube to continuously feed the chemo to my body. Next, I was supplied with a fanny pack that would automatically pump the chemotherapy continuously through my port for sixteen straight weeks. One morning as I arrived in my office, the needle connected to the port burst out, spewing blood and poisonous chemotherapy all over my clothes. I was grateful that it was still very early in the morning, and I was able to leave the office unnoticed. I called my wife to explain the situation as I drove to the clinic. She met me there with clean clothes, and the nurse fixed the needle in the port.

As I adjusted to the medicine pumping through my veins, I was pleasantly surprised that I wasn't experiencing any side effects, although I was more tired than normal. As the doctor added the targeted radiation at week eight, the combination brought on extreme fatigue. I would go to work in the morning, and when I came home in the afternoon, I would pass out, often without eating dinner. I started feeling pain and throbbing in my feet, called neuropathy, from the chemotherapy. As I endured the twice-a-week radiation treatments, it felt like the inner wall of my colon was being shredded into tiny bits. I started experiencing issues with my bowels. I can still remember the fear of losing control over my bodily functions like it was yesterday.

I was not allowed to travel during treatment. As travel was a requirement of my new job, I went into my manager's office and told him about my diagnosis. He had been wondering about the fanny pack. I reassured him that I was committed to doing a good job and would stay focused through my treatment. He was supportive and understanding. During my early days of chemotherapy, some of our friends took my wife and me out on their boat on the lake. It was a hot and humid Nashville day, and beads of sweat dripped down my face. I wanted most to be able to cool off in the water, but with my port and chemo fanny pack, I could only get in up to my thighs. As I took in the view of the lake, questions kept popping into my mind, which distracted me from relaxation. Questions like, *What kind of life will I have if I live?* Then, I would hear laughing, and my focus would shift back to my friends. And then, back to the questions: *Am I going to live? How painful will it be?*

After sixteen weeks, I had an MRI that showed the baseball-sized tumor had shrunk to almost nothing—a huge relief and the goal of the treatment. Because of the location of the tumor and the likelihood that it would come back due to my risk factors, the surgeon removed my entire colon and all my lymph nodes. It was major surgery that lasted for eight hours. I was supposed to be in the hospital for eight days post-surgery, although I was released after four days, probably because I am an overachiever.

A few days after being discharged from the hospital, I went for a follow-up appointment with my oncologist. My surgeon had called and left a message while we were on the way that he had gotten clear margins and that none of the lymph nodes were affected, which meant that my odds were high for surviving. We listened to the message just before going in the office as tears rolled down our cheeks. We each took a deep breath and hugged for what felt like an hour, we were so relieved. When the doctor came into the exam room, she jumped right into explaining different options for the post-surgery chemotherapy. My oncologist was from Russia and had a very factual, unemotional approach to my treatment. About fifteen minutes into the appointment, she stopped and said, "Oh, by the way, the surgeon called and informed me that he got clear margins." Luckily, we had already heard the news, or I would have been a nervous wreck during the appointment.

Following the surgery, I faced adjusting to my new body reality of living with an ostomy. While the transition was quite humbling and challenged my view of myself, it was better than the alternative of dying. As time passed, I became a little more gracious with myself, and it became my new normal. I was a workaholic before my diagnosis, taking my computer to bed at night and working every weekend. After my surgery, I went back to the same grind, always focusing on what I could conquer next at work and dedicating my life to my job. I endured six months of chemotherapy infusions, lasting four to six hours every three weeks. I observed the nurses and watched their caring and attentive nature with each patient, so humble and serving so selflessly.

I would also sit and look around the room, taking in the view of all the other cancer patients like me, imagining some may be facing a worse prognosis than mine. Almost all of them were sleeping, while I worked the entire time with my computer in my lap. I had a high work ethic and continued working, both pre- and post-surgery, for over a year and a half, ending up missing only eight days. Despite my work ethic, my position was eliminated almost immediately after I finished my treatment. While I was able to find another job fairly quickly, I also expanded my focus to include charity work. I started volunteering with a family homeless organization and helped Charlie Kelly, one of the angels mentioned previously, with a colon cancer charity fundraiser called the Blue Note, where I spoke about my experience.

Facing the reality that I could die changed my life forever. The experience forged a deeper bond between my wife and me, growing our love and appreciation for each other. I felt well supported by my friends and was touched to the depths of my soul by how they buoyed and supported me. One standout memory is a party that one of my friends held in my honor. She had everyone sign a picture of a semicolon for me, representing that while cancer is life changing, it was not life ending in my case. It was just a shift to a new normal for me.

My biggest challenge when all the treatment was over was choosing to operate differently at work. I am a very competitive and driven person and had poured myself into my work in the past, prioritizing work above life. Having faced the possibility of dying, I had a new appreciation for the value of my life. I started choosing to leave my computer sooner in the day and spending more time with friends. While my experience was not that long in the past, it feels like a lifetime ago. If I am being honest, some of my workaholic tendencies have slipped back into my work habits lately. I am really looking forward to retirement . . . someday!

My cancer experience also deepened my wife's and my faith. Before the cancer, neither of us had gone to church. We both believed in God, but we didn't celebrate outwardly. After treatment, we started to go to church regularly and my wife started singing in the choir. It gave us a place to feel connected and deepen our faith. We moved to Denver in 2013, and while we have found a supportive community in our neighborhood, we are still searching for a church.

The last time I went to see my oncologist, she said, "You are not going to get colon cancer again, but we pumped a bunch of bad stuff in your body, so you are at a much higher risk of other cancers." *Well great*, I thought, *at least I've walked that road before if I ever face it again.*

Advice for Others

How I supported myself
- I used CaringBridge to update friends and family and share some of my thoughts.
- I never stopped working, although I am not sure that is the best advice.
- I listened to my favorite music.
- I approached each day with gratitude, being appreciative of all that is.
- I did things I enjoyed every day.

How others supported me
- I had someone to guide me through the process and tell me what to expect.
- I had good communication about what was going on.
- Friends supported me in many ways, including sending cards, calling, and coming by to see me.

Helpful tips
- Pay attention to your body and your health—don't put off important screenings.
- There is little that is as important as your health.

- When you know someone who is going through cancer treatment, know it is not typically a death sentence; think about your engagement and keep the friendship going, use humor as you are able, and be present when you visit.
- Encourage conversation about all topics, including how the cancer patient is feeling and what's next in the treatment.
- Always get a second opinion; while I only got one opinion, it is a good idea with the speed at which treatments are changing now.
- Don't get caught up with reading the statistics about cancer—many of the survival rates are scary, but remember that they are averages . . . and you aren't average.
- Don't be afraid to cry.
- Think about what you say to cancer survivors and how it might be received before speaking; one time someone said to me "Oh, at least you don't have a bag," and I actually do have an ostomy, although it is not outwardly noticeable.

PEGGY'S STORY

———— • ● • ————

In was October 2005, and I was in my primary care physician's office for my annual exam. I wasn't having any symptoms. As she was doing the breast exam, we were talking about life and my two daughters. All of a sudden, the flow stopped as she kept her finger on one spot. She looked at me and said, "What is this?" as she pointed to an area on my breast. I replied, "Oh, I have had so many of those." I had learned by then that I have fibrocystic breast tissue and had grown accustomed to having lumps. In the past, I had three lumps that were benign and went away over time. My doctor paused and then said, "Well you should probably get a mammogram. Let's not take any chances." Since this was something I had experienced before, I assumed it was benign and nothing would be wrong, so I took needing a mammogram in a matter-of-fact way. Because of the fibrocystic breast tissue, my doctor also ordered an ultrasound. I didn't share the news with anyone and went on about my day. My doctor's office was able to schedule it within a week since it was a diagnostic mammogram. While the realist in me knew that there could be a problem, I kept an optimistic view and just filed it away. A few months earlier, my sister's seven-year-old daughter had come to live with us for a while, so I was fully focused on life with three girls under the age of fifteen.

Two months earlier in August, my youngest daughter had started fifth grade at a new school. Almost immediately, she met a new friend, and a loving bond formed very quickly. She spoke of him often and how much they had in common. He introduced her to the song "Voice of Truth" by Casting Crowns, which she fell in love with. She played the song around the house as well as in the car, so I soon memorized the words. I fell in love with the comforting truth in the lyrics, and it became one of my favorite songs. How little did I know then that this would become an important thread in the fabric of my life in the very near future.

The week after my doctor's appointment in October, I went by myself to the mammogram appointment, thinking it would be just like my previous experiences. After the technician completed the mammogram and the ultrasound, he said he needed to step out for a minute. I thought someone needed him for something else. He walked back in the room with the radiologist. *Okay, so maybe it is like before and he wants to discuss it with me.* The radiologist introduced himself and said, "I would really like to do a biopsy. Are you able to stay? We can probably get you in pretty quickly." In that moment, it felt like the needle popped off the record on the turntable and everything got real quiet. I could have heard a pin drop. My mind quickly shifted to thinking, *What if this is cancer, what do I know about breast cancer, what are my beliefs?* This was something new to me, as no one close to me had experienced cancer. All of a sudden, I felt peace as one of my favorite songs started playing in my head, giving me a sign that God was with me.

> *But the voice of truth tells me a different story*
> *The voice of truth says, "Do not be afraid!"*
> *The voice of truth says, "This is for My glory"*
> *Out of all the voices calling out to me*
> *I will choose to listen and believe the voice of truth*

Every time I remember that moment, I realize how grateful I was for that song because it gave me comfort, and I knew I wasn't alone. The nurse led me back to a room where I was to wait by myself. They estimated it would take about a half hour. I started flipping through pages of magazines. That is when the fear started to creep in, which is not my normal response. I felt like I was stranded alone on an island. I took some deep breaths to calm my nerves and thought, *This could really be happening*. I played back the events of the past hour and remembered my experience with previous lumps. The doctor had requested more pictures in the past, but not a biopsy. This time was very different. Then I heard:

But the voice of truth tells me a different story. . . .

I was called back for the biopsy shortly after the words played in my head again. It was a pretty straightforward procedure, although time seemed to slow down, and everything around me felt surreal. I am very pragmatic, so I was not overwhelmed with emotion. When I walked out, I remember thinking, *I just had a tissue sample taken that could alter the course of my life. Lord, what do you have in store for me?*

My focus was elsewhere, as I was in the midst of a very stressful back-to-school time. My sister's seven-year-old daughter was living with us while my sister and her husband struggled with some challenging issues. After what started out as a weeklong vacation for my niece, I quickly realized that she needed our warm and comforting family to become her family for an unspecified amount of time, so she stayed with us. We enrolled her in school nearby and now had third-, fifth-, and ninth-grade daughters, each starting the year at new schools. Due to my niece's last-minute enrollment, the only opening was at a neighboring elementary school where I didn't know the faculty, staff, or many of the families. Since my niece had a different last name, and I was her aunt and not her mother, people were curious about her story and almost immediately branded her as different, unsafe, and even damaged. This was heartbreaking to us and something we couldn't control. All we could do was love her and give her a safe, comforting environment. But the struggle existed in our home as well. As we adjusted to our new normal, which included my younger daughter having to share her room, it created a different dynamic in our family that was tricky to navigate. I was grateful to have such a supportive husband through all of this.

A few days after my mammogram and biopsy, I was working part time in a friend's clothing showroom at the Dallas Market Center when my phone rang. I noticed it was my doctor calling, so I stepped outside, knowing that the news would be what I dreaded most. I answered the phone and felt numb and kind of detached as my doctor shared the results. I'm sure she told me the type of cancer, and I'm sure she tried to reassure me that it was *very* treatable, although this was a new realm for me, and fear tried to creep in. I didn't know the language and didn't know the best course of action. I was in uncharted territory and didn't know how I was going to fix this. Then I heard the verse playing in my mind:

But the voice of truth tells me a different story. . . .

As I look back now, I find it odd that I did not pause to try to wrap my mind around this news but instead headed back to work. Was I trying desperately to take a step back in time to what had been my normal? As I stepped foot into the showroom, it was as if the color went out of the room as the words permeated my mind: *Cancer. I have cancer. Cancer is in my body.* My friend saw my face and noticed something was wrong. I said, "My doctor just called and told me I have cancer. She said we caught it early, and it is very slow growing, ductal, hormone fed." My friend came over and hugged me as I continued to sort out the weight of the words I had heard. Then it hit me—my life had now forever changed.

I picked up my phone and dialed my husband's number. "Honey, the doctor just called me. She said it's cancer although it's very treatable." Silence filled the space, and I could almost feel how my words knocked the wind out of him. I knew I needed to be upbeat and added, "We are going to get through this together. It will all work out. No need to worry." But did I believe those words? When I arrived home later that day, we decided to wait until we had more answers before sharing the news with the girls. It was time to go to work and chart my plan of action.

Fortunately, we lived in a city with many highly respected doctors in the breast cancer field, as many women in our community had gone on this journey ahead of me. While several doctors came highly recommended, we chose a man who had a stellar reputation as a world class breast surgeon whom our close friends knew personally. They told us he was guided by a strong faith, which sealed my decision. He graciously agreed to see my husband and me a few days later, late on Friday afternoon. Armed with a fresh yellow pad and pen, we sat with him and got our first lesson on the new language we would learn to speak. We instantly felt a sense of calm from his kind demeanor and began to put our trust in him. He discussed next steps, which included securing an oncologist as well as scheduling surgery to test my lymph nodes. Then he looked at me and said, "If you are going to get breast cancer, this is the type you want. It is slow growing and hormone fed." After he had answered all our questions, his office scheduled the first surgery.

I had the surgery to test the lymph nodes early the following week, and the results came back quickly showing no sign of cancer there. The next step was the mastectomy. We had planned to spend Thanksgiving with my brother and his family in Wimberley. My surgeon assured me that surgery could wait until after Thanksgiving and how important it was to build memories with our family first. Before we left for my brother's house, we sat our girls down and shared the news with them. They had no point of reference, although the word cancer felt scary to them. Without sharing too many details, we told them what my expected treatment was and that I had high odds of a full recovery. We also felt very comfortable telling them that I was not going to die from this if we followed the doctors' recommended treatment plan. A wise friend who had been on this journey recommended that I name people that my girls knew who had successfully battled cancer and were living full lives. So I shared some names with them. They looked at me with surprise and said they never even knew those women had cancer. Hearing this really comforted them and helped them realize this was not a death sentence. Because my younger daughter had a connection to the doctor, I asked them to guess who my doctor was. My surgeon was the dad of her special friend who had introduced her to the song "Voice of Truth." In their young worlds, the only doctors they knew were their orthopedic doctor and their pediatrician. After a few minutes of guessing, I told them the name of my doctor and then said to my youngest daughter, "It's your new friend's dad."

It took her about five seconds to process this before blurting out, "Does that mean that he's seen your boobs?" It was the perfect comic relief!

Treatment Experience

As a cancer patient, I was suddenly popular with an entire team of doctors. One of the doctors on my dream team was a medical oncologist, the one who determines treatment post-surgery. At the time, there was a promising marker that was fast gaining confidence from medical research called the Oncotype DX test. This was a genomic test that analyzed the activity of a group of twenty-one genes from a breast cancer tissue sample that can affect how a cancer is likely to behave and respond to treatment. The Oncotype DX test results assign a recurrence score—a number between zero and one hundred—to the early-stage breast cancer. My doctor used the Oncotype DX test to help figure out my risk of early-stage, estrogen-receptor-positive, HER2-negative breast cancer coming back, as well as how likely I was to benefit from chemotherapy after surgery. The Oncotype DX test was designed to offer more information to help women and their doctors make decisions about chemotherapy. I had a very low score on this test so my oncologist did not add chemotherapy to my treatment, as the side effects would have far outweighed the benefits.

My next step was surgery, which lasted six hours and had two parts. My surgical oncologist performed the mastectomy of my left breast, and then the plastic surgeon came in and performed a latissimus dorsi flap procedure. Recovery from this surgery was tough, as I had never experienced major surgery before. I had two drains and could hardly get out of bed on my own initially. Since I lived as a highly independent woman, this recovery was a crash course in learning how to depend on others and how to ask for help! Life seemed to grind to a halt as I slowly recovered.

My mastectomy was the first part of the reconstruction process. The doctor took a part of my latissimus muscle from my back and brought it around to where the breast's tissue had been removed. An implant would eventually be placed under this muscle but, at the time, an expander was put in its place. The expander was designed to make room for the implant. It was like a balloon filled with liquid, and every month I would return to the plastic surgeon, who added liquid to the expander until it reached the size of the implant. Once that happened, another surgery was scheduled to take out the expander and place the implant, thus completing the reconstruction process. This whole reconstruction process took close to six months. Philippians 1:21 is a verse that comforted me through my healing: "To live is Christ, to die is gain." My husband didn't like the "to die" part. Following my single mastectomy, I was put on Tamoxifen for five years as insurance to reduce the risk that the cancer would come back in the future.

In October of 2008, three years later, I went in for my annual checkup. My doctor said, "I'm not supposed to release you until after five years, but all indications are that this journey is behind you." *Woo-hoo, I beat this, I am done!* I thought. For all intents and purposes, I felt no lingering effects from my cancer. I was on the Tamoxifen but was having no side effects from it. I was quickly subsumed into my busy life. However, two short months later, in January 2009, I found a small lump just under the skin of the same breast that had the mastectomy. My doctor ordered a biopsy and it came back positive for the same type of cancer. *How could this be?* I had been told I had a 2 percent chance of recurrence, which is lower than the chance that an average woman has in contracting breast cancer! My dream team of doctors was more shocked than I was that it came back. "Not you, Peggy. You were done." *How in the world could this happen?* I wondered.

My doctor explained that it just takes one breast cell left behind from the mastectomy for cancer to grow. This must have been what happened. He did a lumpectomy to remove the lump, and then he recommended I have radiation treatments for six weeks. It was also evident that the Tamoxifen had not worked for me. Because my cancer was hormone fed, the doctor wanted to rid my body of as many hormones as possible. I had surgery to remove my ovaries, which accelerated menopause. I was then put on Arimadex, which is the post-menopausal equivalent of Tamoxifen, a hormone inhibitor. No one prepared me for the roller coaster ride I would go on with the removal of hormones from my body. Who knew how our emotions were tied to hormones? Not me! It was a crazy out-of-body experience that would take nine months of prescribed antidepressants to bring me back to equilibrium. Not wanting to be a burden to anyone, I shouldered much of this later journey by myself. I didn't want to scare my kids or overburden my husband. I went to my daily radiation treatments alone because, after all, I was a strong independent woman. *Why drag someone else into this? I got this.* I remember seeing so many others at radiation who were clearly fighting for their lives. Some lost their battle, as I never saw them return. I was grateful I was fighting a form of the disease that was more burdensome than life threatening.

In 2017, I had been on Arimadex for nine years and received the blessing to stop taking it. After getting off the drug, I was surprised at the sense of relief that I felt. I hadn't realized I was still carrying a cancer burden around with me. While this cancer experience has taught me many things, one powerful lesson is how important my health is. I am much more aware of my body now.

Advice for Others

How I supported myself

- I prayed daily and kept the song "The Voice of Truth" close in my heart.
- I wrote about my story on a CaringBridge site—it was an easy way to inform everyone, and writing about my story helped me heal; the comments and scripture that friends and family wrote gave me strength and courage to carry on.

How others supported me

- Several friends came over and planted new flowers in our beds.
- My husband and I would get together with five other couples to pray—it was really powerful for me to see men getting on their knees and praying, knowing that I was the recipient of the prayers.
- I felt more uplifted than ever when I was going through the treatment, as if loving arms from my friends and family were wrapped all around me.
- A close friend told me that if I had to go through chemotherapy infusions and would lose my hair, she would cut her hair so I could use it to make a wig.

Helpful tips

- Make a list of survivors who appear normal and share the names.
- Find a mantra or song that is uplifting and will carry you through; mine was "The Voice of Truth".
- If you believe, look for God at work in the journey, because God is working!
- Know that cancer is a roller coaster ride for the patient, and chemotherapy drugs hinder the patient's ability to remember much of anything; a journal is a helpful gift so the patient can keep track of details and symptoms.

Surprising experiences

On my CaringBridge site, I got an email from a woman who wrote: "I had a friend who directed me to your CaringBridge site. Not knowing you, I thought this was a strange request, but I was curious, so I pulled up your site. I live a few blocks away, and we happen to go to your same church. I was raised with a strong faith, and it was always a big part of my identity. Last year, I was pregnant, and my husband and I were thrilled at the thought of beginning our family! Tragically, we lost our baby in a miscarriage, and I was devastated! *Why would God let this happen?* I was angry at God and suddenly all of His promises I had relied on to sustain me up to this point just faded away. I ran away from God and the church for many months. I didn't understand any of it and was bitter, angry, and heartbroken. But then something happened. As I read through the many scripture-filled posts on your CaringBridge site, which were meant to encourage and support you and your family in this battle, I was reminded of God's attributes and promises. My stone-cold heart began to melt as I was bathed in these words that were so familiar to me. God is so mysterious; he used your cancer journey to draw me back to Him and to begin my healing process!" What a gift this was for me. God used my journey to bring back a lost sheep. In my broken, diseased body, God used my journey for His Glory. Wow! Just *wow!*

ROBERT O'S STORY

———•—●—•———

It was early January 2008 when I noticed something wasn't right. I had retired from the fire department a few years before and was working part time as a painting contractor. One day when I went to the bathroom, I noticed some blood in the toilet. I didn't pay much attention as I just thought I had strained myself climbing up a ladder, since I was sixty-one. Or maybe I strained it playing softball. Either way, I filed it away and didn't say anything. My wife and I lived on five acres of land, and taking care of the property kept me busy. Our morning routine was to wake up, drink our coffee in bed, and watch the morning news. One of these mornings when I went to go to the bathroom, I wasn't able to urinate anymore, and I noticed some throbbing pain. I walked back in the bedroom and said, "Honey, I am not able to pee."

She looked at me and said, with a concerned voice, "We need to go to the ER then." I told her no, and she said yes. If you know me, you know my wife is always right. Pretty soon she was driving me to the ER.

We arrived at the ER and they took me back pretty quickly. We lived in a small town and it was not a busy morning for the ER. The doctor examined me and had the nurse start a catheter to relieve the pain. I immediately felt better. The doctor explained that I probably had an overactive bladder and prescribed some medicine. He also wrote down the name of a urologist and recommended I make an appointment. We left, and I called the urologist on the way home. I had been healthy all of my sixty-one years so far, and I trusted doctors to know what was wrong and what to do to help me. I continued experiencing the urination problems and pain for the next several months. It happened two to three times a week, and I would go to the urologist's office during the week or the ER on the weekend. My wife would question me from time to time, and I would say, "I am sure everything is okay. I am going to a doctor, and he is supposed to know what to do."

By the middle of May, I was still having the symptoms and decided something might be wrong. I went in for an appointment with the urologist. After he examined me, he pulled out a cystoscope, a thin tube with a light at the end. He was looking at a screen as he used the scope. And that is when he saw it, the lesion in my bladder. He said, "Robert, there is a lesion in your bladder. It doesn't look like anything to worry about. I'm taking a sample and will send it out for pathology. I will be in touch soon with the results." The last thing I wanted to think about was something wrong. I was still in denial and believed that this was just old age.

Several weeks later, my doctor called and asked me to come in the office to discuss the test results. I called my wife at work and she said she would meet me there. It was June 6th, my wife's birthday. The minute we saw each other, I said, "I'm scared."

She replied, "Me too." We each took a deep breath, almost in unison, grabbed each other's hand, and went inside.

The doctor didn't waste any time getting to the point. He simply said, "You have bladder cancer, and it has metastasized." As these harsh words started to permeate my mind, I felt like I had been punched in the face. I leaned back and opened my eyes wider, as if that would change the words; then I took a deep, gasping breath. When I made eye contact with my wife, she could see the fear in my eyes, something that was a first in our many years of marriage. My wife says she can still see the picture of my reaction in her mind, as if it just happened.

I started to question why this was happening to me. All of a sudden, my life had changed forever. I had so many questions. I really didn't know what was going on. My family was very supportive and helpful, which kept me going day by day. The urologist planned to refer me to one team of doctors, although the wait for an appointment was a month. I was anxious to move forward and have a plan as quickly as I could. One of the office staff was able to get me into an academic medical center, a few hours away, within two weeks. I went in with an open mind. When I arrived for my appointment, I learned I was meeting with the head of bladder cancer research and several other doctors. I felt fully supported to have a team of doctors on my case and working to figure out a plan quickly.

The oncologist started asking me regular questions, such as did I drink alcohol or smoke. I said, "Yes, I chew tobacco and drink beer."

The oncologist looked at me and said, in a very matter-of-fact way, "Well, you don't anymore."

I really didn't want to give up my vices and tried to negotiate with him, "Can we barter here a little and you take one and I keep one?" He seemed to be getting a little annoyed with me at this point and gave it to me straight, right between the eyes. He asked, "Do you want to live? If so, then no more drinking or chewing tobacco." I walked out of the building and threw away my chewing tobacco.

My wife looked at me with surprise and said, "Wow, you are really going to do this?"

I replied, "You bet your ass I am!"

The oncologist ordered several additional tests and a biopsy. The next day, he told me I had stage IV bladder cancer and recommended I start with chemotherapy and then have surgery. Given the severity of my situation, I was to have infusions three times a week for eight weeks. When you mention stage IV cancer to anyone, fear wells up in their minds, and they imagine it is a death sentence. For me, it was not the stage of the cancer that I was concerned about. I was more angered that something foreign was in my body. My wife was transparent with what was going on all along the way, which was really helpful. I asked her early on in my treatment, "Do me a favor and don't patronize me. Tell me the truth, always. I need you to keep me upbeat and positive, and I don't want to see your pouty face. I will think something else is wrong. Tell me exactly what is going on when you know something, or my mind will know you are hiding something from me."

The oncologist wanted me to start as soon as possible. He told me to go up to the third floor, the oncology floor, and schedule my chemotherapy infusions. I was still struggling with the question, *Why me?* I was feeling sorry for myself. When I stepped off the elevator on the third floor, I turned left and saw all the pediatric patients with tumors, young children who were worse off than me. Watching their faces and imagining that their lives might be cut short before ever starting got me over my pity party really quickly. I decided not to feel sorry for myself, as I knew many of these kids were not going to live to see all that I have seen. I went and told my wife, "I am over feeling sorry for myself." It is amazing how God showed me what I needed to see in that moment.

Treatment Experience

Given the late stage of my cancer, I started chemotherapy infusions the following week and would go in every Wednesday from eight until five, Thursday from noon until five, and Friday from two until five. My doctor recommended a drug regimen called MVAC, which is a combination of four chemotherapy drugs, and I would get a Neulasta shot on Fridays to help boost my immune system. I followed this routine for three weeks on and then rested one week, then three weeks on again and rest. I endured this treatment for eight weeks from June through August 2006. Before I finished my last round, my oncologist recommended I go forward with the surgery. The surgery was scheduled for September 11, and since I was a retired fire fighter, my wife and I talked about whether that would be a good thing or a bad thing, in view of the tragic event in the US on September 11, 2001. We decided it was a good thing.

The oncologist called my wife to explain my surgery and check on us due to the tropical storm. I endured an eleven-hour surgery to remove my bladder and reconstruct a bladder out of my lower colon. When I was in the hospital, it was the fastest ten days of my life. My pain was managed by a morphine pump. Two days before I was to be discharged after the surgery, my incision became infected and the nurse had to reopen it to clean it out, and then put a new bandage on it. My wife sat down, feeling queasy from what she was watching. She looked at the nurse and said, "I can't do this."

The nurse replied, "You can do this, and you will do this." During my ten days, I had nurses come by and have lunch in my room to check in on me. The physical therapist came in two days after surgery and said, "I am going to get you up to walk tomorrow." I was planning to try to convince him not to. The next day, the nurse came by and said Chris, the physical therapist, was on his way. Chris came to my room and stood as tall as the door. He looked at me and said, in a very positive voice, "Are you ready to walk?"

His presence changed my mind. I replied, "How far?" Given his size and determination, I knew there was no hope of talking him out of walking that day.

Post-surgery, I started chemotherapy infusions at the end of October for four months. I decided I was going to stick around to kick up more dust. Even though it was a "mild" chemo, I did not tolerate it well. My blood counts were often too low to allow me to get the infusion. In the beginning of February 2009, the oncologist said, "Robert, I think your body is telling us it's had enough chemo. I think we should stop." He ordered a scan and in March 2009, we found out I was "disease free." There are no words to describe what either one of us felt at that time. Relief—obviously—thankful, grateful, but still guarded. It took me six to eight months to fully recover. During the treatment and surgery, I lost fifty pounds. At the one-year mark, my nurse said, "Mr. Bob, we need to put weight on you."

I replied, "You go tell that doctor that I need my beer." She did, and the doctor agreed to let me start drinking beer again.

For five years, I went back for tests every six months to make sure I was still in remission. I was overwhelmed by the kindness and top-notch care I received from my physicians at the center. This experience has taught me so much, including when to seek care. Now, every time I feel something that isn't right, I get it checked out. I am able to go to the firefighter clinic for retirees and get a B-12 shot once a month. I now know that if the first urologist had examined me with the scope in the beginning, he would have found the lesion early, and I likely would have been able to keep my bladder and prostate. Based on my experience, I will now question a doctor if I am having symptoms and do not feel that I am being fully examined or if my issues are not being addressed.

About a month before each appointment, I would get antsy and worried about what the doctor might discover. After the appointment, I would be relieved. When we left the doctor's office after my final follow-up appointment five years later, my wife and I were both quiet. She asked me, "How do you feel about being 'cut loose'?"

I looked at her and said, "Actually, it makes me scared. No one is watching anymore. The responsibility has shifted from someone with authority and intelligence checking me out regularly to being back on my own. It's now up to me to take care of myself—I feel left all alone and need to grab myself by the seat of my pants." She and I both agreed we were apprehensive about losing the security blanket. It was a happy day on the one hand and a very scary day on the other.

At first, there was a question about whether I would live or die. I felt sorry for myself and wondered, *Why me?* I had lots of people praying for me, and I believe in the power of prayer, although I don't preach the gospel. I encourage others to be careful with their choices. I talk about my experience to most everyone who will listen, rather than giving advice to others about what they should do. Every person's body is different. While I have always had a strong marriage, this experience definitely strengthened our relationship. We now pray together every afternoon, just before dinner. We thank God for answering our prayers, and we pray for others. This is something we never took the time to do before my diagnosis. It is also important to consider that advancements in cancer treatment are happening every day. If you know of someone with a recent diagnosis, imagine that they will survive it and go support them.

Advice for Others

How I supported myself
- Stayed focus on getting better, maintained a good, positive attitude, and had a strong will to live.
- I tried to keep a sense of normalcy in everyday life, no pity parties.

How others supported me
- My wife, family and friends stayed upbeat and positive to keep me upbeat and positive.

Helpful tips
- Help others hold a positive space; imagine the possibilities rather than focusing on what is wrong.
- If you are having symptoms, go to a big medical practice or academic medical center where they keep up with medical advances.

- Trust your gut—my wife didn't have a good feeling about the first doctor.
- Don't go it alone, but welcome and invite in a support system; when you know you are covered in prayer, everything changes for the better.

HOLLY'S STORY

Given the history of breast cancer in my family, I started having annual mammograms at a young age. In October of 2008, I received a normal mammogram report. Our Christmas that year was like any other, spending time with our family and with friends. We enjoyed fancy home-cooked dinners and hosted a party where we served s'mores for the neighborhood kids. Our dogs were young at the time, so we put little reindeer antler headbands with Christmas lights on them. Santa brought lots of fun gifts for my daughter, including a cat suit, an American Girl doll, and a Wii. We all spent many hours playing Dance Dance Revolution. As New Year's Eve came, the normalcy of the holiday vanished when I discovered a lump in my breast. I found it by accident as we were going to sleep. I remember exclaiming to my husband, "What the heck is this?" It was pretty large, about the size of a marble. I'd had cysts before, so I tried to focus on it being another one of those until I could get it checked out. Even thinking about that time now makes my stomach drop. The doctor's office was closed, so I tried not to think about it until I could call for an appointment. However, looking back at the photos from the holiday, I can see the fear in my eyes.

When my close friend came to town later that day, I confided in her, "Hey, so I found a lump in my breast. I'm hoping it's just a cyst like I've had before." She wrapped her arms around me as I sat with the words that filled my thoughts. *I found something in my breast. Could it be cancer? I don't want to believe it.* My friend and her husband started praying for me right away without my even asking, which gave me comfort.

Since Friday was a holiday, I called the women's breast center the following Monday and was able to get an appointment the next day for tests. I did my best to keep distracted and not think about the lump. I went alone, still trying to focus on it being a cyst. The lump still did not show on the mammogram. The technician told me I needed an ultrasound. This still was not that alarming, because I always had to have ultrasounds after a mammogram. I even told the technician I thought it was probably a cyst, but her lack of response made me think maybe it was not a cyst as I had been hoping. As I sat in the waiting room, I called my Bible study friend and asked for prayers. At some point, the clinic called the breast cancer patient support person to come sit with me. Then we went in to hear the news. The radiologist said, "This is highly suspicious of cancer, although we will need a biopsy to know for sure." I felt my stomach drop, and my heart started beating twice as fast as I processed this reality, my greatest fear coming true. I thanked the doctor and left, still in shock from what she had said.

I knew taking action would help me feel like I was in control. I decided to go to an oncologist in the medical center in Houston where my dad had worked as a physician and taught at the medical school. My mother still lived in Houston and had a compassionate and helpful oncologist from her journey with breast cancer, who was also a friend of my dad's. I was able to get in right away for an appointment with him—I pretty much told him on the phone that I was getting in the car and heading his way from Austin. When I arrived, we met briefly, and he was able to schedule a biopsy right away. Following the biopsy, I shifted my focus to the waiting game, which felt like walking through knee-deep water.

Before I found the lump, I had planned to go away to a women's retreat at Laity Lodge with my long-time Bible study sisters the second weekend in January. I was questioning whether I should still go, as I was waiting for biopsy results. My friends convinced me that the retreat was exactly what I needed, so we headed to the Texas Hill Country. The weekend filled my heart and soul with comfort, and I was able to distract myself somewhat from the worry of what the test results might show. I was surrounded by supportive women who let me talk about my fears and prayed over me the last morning; we also enjoyed heartfelt fellowship, worship, and laughter. One unusually warm morning we hiked over to the beautiful swimming hole and decided to jump in, even though it was January. My sisters said we needed to swim in the healing waters of the blue hole, but we did not have our suits. We decided to swim anyway, sans bathing suits. What we didn't know at the time was that an older couple was staying up the hill at the quiet house overlooking the swimming hole—they had hiked down the back trail and had seen us swimming. This story spread like wildfire through the lodge, and as it was retold over time, acquired a new ending: The next day, the older man said to his wife, "Honey, we should take another hike to the blue hole!" It still makes me laugh when I think of that.

I returned to Austin, feeling buoyed by the women and my time in nature, although still anxious about the results I was waiting to hear. When they were ready, I drove back to Houston. My oncologist gave me the news I had been dreading. He said, "Holly, the test results do show cancer. You found it early, as it is stage I, and it's called mucinous carcinoma, which is an invasive type of cancer." He explained more details and said I would need additional tests to make sure it had not spread. He had said he thought I would need a lumpectomy, until some suspicious spots showed up on the new scans.

I felt a mastectomy would give me the highest chance of eliminating a recurrence, given my family history of breast cancer, although I was open to waiting until we knew more. While tests did not show any spread in my body, there would be no definitive answer until the sentinel biopsy at the time of surgery. I felt so frightened not knowing for sure. I was determined to eliminate the chance of recurrence, regardless of its impact on me. I felt overwhelmed with all the unknowns and all the information gathering that was still before me to best determine the type of procedure and which surgeon to use.

I work in the research field, which was both a blessing and a curse. I quickly started an in-depth research process to learn more details about the type of surgery, whether to do a nipple sparing surgery or not, and to evaluate whether breast implants or a flap procedure would be best for me. I obsessively gathered information and talked to countless people in the process. I was surprised that so many acquaintances and doctors told me what to do instead of simply explaining what they had done or giving me options to consider. One of my great blessings was to have my husband, close friends, and dedicated oncologist to work through options with me as partners in the process, going over pros and cons and understanding all the ramifications.

During this process, I realized it was time to activate my strong support system of friends and prayer groups. In the midst of my fear and concern over what might happen, having prayer groups and friends supporting me helped me feel like I was not alone. A close friend also started an email chain to share updates, especially while I was in the hospital, which felt so supportive and loving. My husband would send her updates that she would share via email with the group. We could easily give her another email address to add, and having a single point of contact simplified communications in such a helpful way.

I met with a surgeon in Houston first, as my father had worked in that medical center his entire adult life and wanted me to have surgery there. We were still considering a lumpectomy because the other results were not in yet. The surgeon said, "Holly, do you realize how close your tumor is to the chest wall? Most surgeons would not be aggressive enough to make sure they get all the cancer, but I will be." This really scared me, because he seemed to be worried that the cancer had invaded my chest wall. I left the office and drove back to Austin. Once I learned that a mastectomy would be better for me given the additional results, I met with a surgeon in Austin. This surgeon actually left me in tears because he was so negative about flap procedures and insisted I go with an implant. I was extremely concerned about implants and decided I wanted more input; I sought advice from an expert who no longer practiced medicine and served as an advisor to women with breast cancer. I shared my concerns and mistrust of implants, and he shared research indicating that, in fact, there were issues with implants, and some had even been linked to other types of cancer.

While I was concerned with aesthetics during the time, I also felt afraid of what my prognosis would be. I had decided that I preferred a free flap reconstruction to breast implants, and I continued my research to find a surgeon who was comfortable performing this type of procedure. I found one such surgeon in Houston, but she was out of the country for several months on a speaking tour. I was not able to find a surgeon in Austin who performed the free flap procedure in 2009. Thanks to one of my dearest friends who works in the medical community and who later in the process did my tattooing for me, I was able to find an entire surgical group in San Antonio that focused on this type of reconstruction after breast cancer. I was thrilled with this connection, especially as the practice was so close to where I lived.

I made an appointment with the surgeon in San Antonio. As I was sharing my plans with my friend, she said, "How about I come with you and take notes? We can talk about what we each heard on the drive back." I was delighted with her offer of support and felt relieved that I would have her with me. I was still sorting out the reality that I had cancer and was grateful to have an extra set of ears to help me process things. We drove to the appointment, and when the surgeon came in the exam room, I remember feeling the tight hold of worry and fear began to loosen. He was compassionate and confident, and I knew I was in good and extremely competent hands. When I learned that faith was a big part of this surgeon and his partner's practice, it confirmed for me that I was in the right place. With great relief, I relaxed, knowing that my decision was made and a large part of my work was done. All I had to do was to put myself in the hands of this doctor, who I believe was an answer to my prayers, and do what he recommended. The surgeon made me laugh when he said, "Holly, I don't think you have enough fat on your stomach for this procedure." He had me turn around to see if a gluteal flap would work and he said, "Oh yeah, we can make you a double D." We decided that I would likely need the gap flap procedure because I had more excess fat on my bottom than on my stomach. My friend reminded me of some questions I had forgotten to ask, and the surgeon sat with us, patiently answering all of them. As we drove back and discussed the details, I realized that she had heard things I didn't remember hearing, likely due to the stress of the situation. I decided that I would make sure to have someone with me at any future appointments.

Treatment Experience

I decided to have the mastectomy and gluteal flap procedure at the same time, which was a seven-hour surgery. My surgeon went out of his way to explain all the details of what would happen next, making the process easier for me and my family. Before I was wheeled back to surgery, he prayed with me. He had a very unassuming demeanor and was quite humble about his amazing gift and talent as a surgeon. I went into surgery feeling at ease that I was in good hands, all would go well, and I would make it through.

I was a little nervous due to the length of surgery and anesthesia so, just in case, I had made a video for my sweet daughter. The surgeon did the sentinel biopsy during the surgery. After the procedure, I spent a week in the hospital. It was a tough recovery; I felt completely vulnerable and yet strangely calm, as I felt closer to God than I had ever been. My dad and stepmom came for the surgery, and my mom came and stayed in San Antonio with my daughter all week, entertaining her and doing fun things like going to Sea World.

The day before I was to be released, my daughter was planning to come see me for the first time. She was all dressed up and excited about seeing me, but just before she and my mom got there, the flap failed. The doctors had monitored the pulse rate and oxygenation of the flap just like a newborn infant in the NICU. I was immediately prepped and rushed into surgery. My surgeon was out of town, but his partner was able to identify and remove a tiny clot that was blocking blood flow and oxygen to my reconstructed breast. The clot was likely due to a respiratory therapist not knowing the type of surgery I had experienced. He had directed me to place a pillow over my breast and cough. This happened the one time that my husband stepped away to get some food, and I was left alone. I had tried to argue with the therapist, but I was still groggy from the pain medication and finally did as he requested. And while this extra surgery led me to stay another week in the hospital, I continued to gain strength and didn't experience any other surprises. Before I left the hospital, the sentinel node results came in, and we were overjoyed to learn that the cancer had not spread. I felt the tightened muscles on my neck start to relax as the fear transitioned to belief that I would survive.

Whenever I tried to thank my surgeon and compliment him on how well everything had turned out, he would look at me with a smile and say, "All the glory goes to God who guides my hands." I had the surgery over spring break in March 2009, and my recovery took about a month. My doctor prescribed Tamoxifen post-surgery since my type of cancer was hormone receptor positive. I went back to living my life with the plan that someday I would have a preventative mastectomy with the same reconstruction on my right side, although I had not set a date.

That someday arrived just as my life had returned to normal and I had put cancer out of my mind. I went in for my annual scans in March of 2010, and something showed up in my right breast. I was catapulted right back into that state of fear. Three different spots were found, some on an MRI and some on a mammogram. I did all the testing in Houston under my oncologist's direction. We did punch and needle biopsies; the needle biopsy was mammogram guided. During this biopsy, I had to lie on my stomach on a gurney with an opening at breast level. The radiologist and technicians were down under the gurney, performing the biopsy. The biopsy was painful; I could not move at all for quite some time due to the imaging. I closed my eyes and prayed that it was not cancer and imagined that Jesus was holding me instead of the table.

I got dressed after the procedure and headed back to Austin, still sore and in pain. I was so hoping this time was not cancer and then my oncologist called. He said, "Holly, I am sad to say the tumors are malignant. I would recommend you have the same surgery as you did on your left side. We caught it early, so there is no need for chemotherapy or radiation." I was devastated with this news as fear filled my mind. I took several deep breaths and realized this time would be different. I already had a surgeon and knew what type of surgery I wanted. And I had experienced it once. As I sat still thinking about this, the fear started to dissolve into faith, as I believed I would survive. I called my surgeon and scheduled an appointment. When I arrived with my friend, it felt so reassuring to be back in my surgeon's presence, as he was so compassionate and highly competent. I went into the hospital in April of 2010 for a right-side mastectomy and reconstruction. My surgeon prayed with me before I went under anesthesia. After the surgery, I stayed in the hospital for a week to recover, similar to before. This time, I had someone with me the entire time and experienced no issues.

I prepared several things for my daughter before my first surgery in case I didn't survive. I wrote her letters in her journal. I talked to my best friends—my daughter's godmother, her aunt and "aunties," and each of my sister friends—and assigned them each future jobs, such as helping my daughter pick out her wedding dress, and mainly never letting her forget how much I loved her. I imagine it sounds a little dramatic, but I didn't know if the cancer had spread yet and wanted to prepare for the worst. My family and friends absolutely promised that if the worst happened, which it probably wouldn't, they would always be there for my daughter, on each birthday, special occasion, and all her life.

Whenever my surgeon came by to check on me, I would try to thank him, and he as usual would give all the glory to God. I felt deeply grateful for how he shepherded me and my family through what turned out to be a lengthy process. My surgeon and his partners made an extremely difficult time in my life much easier for us. I am eternally grateful to them for carrying me through this time and for bringing some levity, making it not so scary, and giving me a sense of normalcy and hope.

As I reflect on our entire journey, I remember how terrified and worried about possible outcomes my husband and I were. Through our experience, my husband and I became closer; he was at my side through every step. Also, and most importantly, we had never felt so close to God; all we could do was rely on Him. He used this time to strengthen our faith and to teach us over and over that He is always with us and will never fail us, especially when outcomes are unknown and times are hard. God also used us to strengthen others' faith as well. Throughout the journey, we had so many friends and family members praying for us, and we prayed so much that our faith was apparent to others. My husband kept making me CDs with a particular set of my favorite Jesus tunes on them for my MRI appointments, and I kept giving them away to the technicians. The nurses in the hospital noticed our faith and said they were inspired by it. God used my journey with cancer to achieve His ends of bringing all of us close to Him.

Since February of 2019, I have been seeing an Austin-based oncologist who came highly recommended after my oncologist in Houston passed away. She shared with me some new research indicating that, while I thought I was past the window for a potential recurrence at five years and now almost ten years out, apparently there is a recurrence risk to twenty years and beyond for the hormone-fed type of breast cancer I had. As such, I remain diligent about self-exams and annual scans.

Advice for Others

How I supported myself
- I took time off from work for a month to give myself space to heal and did not have many guests at first; just my family, including my mom, and a few close friends.
- I learned the value of life and was grateful every day for another day.
- I prayed and talked to God *all* the time, and I learned that being fearful can be quieted by this and by praising Him.

How others supported me
- The experience gave me new respect for my husband and how supportive and strong he is.
- A friend came and stayed with us after the second procedure, made us dinners, and took care of our daughter.
- Two different friends went with me to appointments as I was talking to surgeons; they kept me company and would take notes and remind me of questions, and then we would discuss what we heard on the drive back, which was so helpful.
- I was blessed with countless prayer groups who buoyed me and made a huge difference; my mom's Bible study and the

church's entire prayer team, along with my Bible study sisters and countless other friends were praying and sending cards.

- Along with my family, my dear friend from school and her husband traveled to San Antonio to pray over me and with me before my second surgery and wrote passages and prayers down for me for me to read if I was anxious.
- A dear friend of over twenty years, who is an aesthetician, tattooed my nipples for me and made me feel completely whole again.
- This friend, her big strapping husband, as well as my daughter's godmother, my cousins, and all the grandparents attended my daughter's dance recital and brought her flowers while I was in the hospital.

Helpful tips
- There have been so many advancements in the cancer field that I recommend if you or someone you love has been diagnosed, you approach the discovery process with an open mind, as so much can be done today.
- Be diligent with scans and self-exams and know your body—it saved my life.
- If you know someone who has been diagnosed with cancer, I would recommend listening, being compassionate, talking about options, and if it applies, even sharing what you chose to do, but understand the choice of treatment is up to that person.
- If someone you love is hospitalized, be in the hospital room with that person to advocate for them at all times.

NIKKI'S STORY

———— • ● • ————

On a mild Colorado night in late June 2014, I was lying in bed watching TV, trying to relax so I could fall asleep. I could hear my husband breathing soundly next to me, as he had fallen asleep. I had my hands on my chest and, all of a sudden, my pinky finger touched something on my right breast. I thought, *Hmmm, what can this be?* It was during the time of month when I was menstruating, and my breasts were fibrocystic anyway, meaning I had felt rope-like bumps before that would come and go. This lump felt a little bigger than any I had felt before, about the size of a pea. I decided it was nothing, filing the discovery away and dozing off to sleep.

A week later, I remembered the lump and decided to see if it was still there. As I ran my index finger over the area, I could still feel it. I asked my husband, "Honey, would you come feel this for me? I found a lump." He stopped what he was doing and came over, agreeing that I should get it checked out. I reached for my phone and called to make an appointment with my primary care doctor, successfully scheduling one for the next day. I went in for the appointment, still imagining that it was nothing. My doctor came in the exam room and after examining me, said, "Nikki, I think it would be good to have this evaluated further. I am going to write an order for a mammogram." My mind starting racing as

I thought, *Okay, so now this is more than just dense tissue forming lumps. There must be something wrong. What's going to happen next? Do I have cancer? Will I lose my hair?* I was more concerned about what I would have to go through if it was cancer. I wasn't afraid of the cancer, as I had endured a life-threatening brain procedure just a few short months before.

When I got home, I told my husband about the mammogram. He said, "Let's take this one day at a time. It's just a scan for now. We'll get through it together." Given my recent health experience, I no longer feared for my life, but I worried about my seven-year-old son and the impact on him if something was wrong.

A few days later, I went to the imaging center for a diagnostic mammogram. The technician called me back pretty quickly and started taking images of my right breast. She finished the standard images, looked at them, and then came over and said, "Um, I need to take a few more pictures." Since I worked in a doctor's office, I instinctively knew this was a sign that something wasn't right. My mind started racing ahead again: *What if this is cancer?* The technician took the pictures and then had me sit in the waiting room by the large fish tank, while she went to talk to the radiologist. She came out fifteen minutes later and called me back, letting me know that I needed an ultrasound. As we walked to the room, she could probably see the concern on my face. As we got settled in the ultrasound room, she shared that she had been diagnosed with cancer before. She looked like she was in her twenties. It distracted me a little to think about her and what that must have felt like at such a young age. Before I knew it, she was finished and said she would go share the results with the radiologist and be back soon. As I sat there staring at the tan wall, my stomach started turning over as I felt in my gut that this lump was cancer. I focused intently on the magazine I was flipping through, zeroing in on the details of each picture and story.

The technician came back with the radiologist in about fifteen minutes. He introduced himself and said, "Nikki, this spot looks concerning. The next step is for you to have a biopsy. I know this is tough news to hear; do you any questions for me?" He explained what would happen next and then left. The technician waited for me and walked me out to the front desk. I was able to schedule the biopsy for two days later. I tried to distract myself as I waited the two days, focusing on my son and his busy summer schedule. I ended up going in by myself for the biopsy, as my dad was having prostate cancer treatment, and my husband was at work. I met the radiologist and he started the biopsy, which was ultrasound-guided, first by numbing my breast and then snipping off samples of tissue. He took a couple of samples and kept going. All of a sudden, he was mid-breast and clipped a nerve, as I felt a shot of pain all the way up to my shoulder. My body flinched and I winced as tears started pouring down my cheeks. He looked at me and said, "Did you feel that?"

"Yes!" I cried. He numbed it some more to get the last sample, and then finished. As I drove home, I started to feel chills racing up and down my spine, wondering what would happen to my son and how he would take it if this was cancer.

As I waited for the results, I tried to distract myself by cleaning the house, doing laundry, and taking care of my son. Several days later, on July 22, I was home alone when my phone rang at ten in the morning. That moment is forever etched in my memory. I was standing in the kitchen washing dishes. I answered the phone and heard the doctor say, "Nikki, I'm sorry. The results came back, and you do have cancer. We caught it early, which is good."

As the doctor started to say what would happen next, I replied, "Okay, okay," not hearing what she was saying.

She said, "I am going to hang up now, because I don't think you are absorbing this news."

"Okay!" I said and hung up. My mind quickly shifted to thinking, *What I want most is a cigarette. You are dumb ass—that is probably what caused the cancer. Oh, and I have it anyway, so does it matter?* I grabbed a cigarette and went outside, lighting it, and sorting out the news I just heard. I was pacing in our backyard as I smoked, wondering what would happen next. I pulled out my phone and called my husband, "Hey, the doctor just called, and the lump tested positive for breast cancer. She said I need to pick an oncologist, and they would take it from there. I am going to use Dad's oncologist, because I really like her."

My husband replied, "We'll do what we've got to do, and you will be fine, Nikki. It will all work out." What I wanted most in this moment was sweet compassion and to be comforted, although I didn't ask for it.

I hung up from my husband and called my dad's oncologist to make an appointment. I was approaching the time in late July when my left hip surgery was scheduled. And now I had cancer. I was becoming an expert on navigating a healthcare system I didn't care to know this personally. A few days later, when I was meeting with my oncologist, she said, "The good news is, you found the lump early. We will do surgery. You have the option of going through chemotherapy and radiation. It's really up to you. The Tamoxifen should take care of anything remaining."

I took a deep breath, as one of my fears was losing my long, straight hair. Then I looked at her and said, "So I am scheduled to have hip surgery next week. Which surgery am I doing first?"

She said, "I would go ahead with the hip surgery first, as it will be an easier procedure. Plus, you have to quit smoking at least six weeks before the mastectomy and reconstructive surgery, or the skin over your implant won't heal." She continued to talk about what kind of surgery I wanted and offered to try a lumpectomy. Since I had tested positive for the BRCA2 gene, I decided to be aggressive and have a double mastectomy. I left the office with a plan for next steps and stopped by the neighborhood pharmacy on the way home. I was determined to be able to move forward with the surgery as soon as possible and bought a patch to quit smoking. I had stopped smoking when I went through my brain experience and had started again only a few months before.

I made it to my hip surgery the following week, in late July, anxious to move forward so I could get this foreign mass of cancer out of my body. The surgery went well, and I was moved to a room for an overnight stay. When the nurse came by to complete her rounds, she introduced herself and told me she was going to try to get me up to go to the bathroom. As she walked up next to the bed, she said, "So, what are you going to do with this new hip?"

I was still groggy from the anesthesia and feeling a little numb. I replied, "I am going to go get my boobs cut off, I have cancer."

She looked startled at my matter-of-fact response and said, "Oh, I wouldn't even know what a lump was if I had one."

I was becoming so used to being poked and prodded in all parts of my body that my modesty had disappeared. "Well here, you can feel it. Here it is, a lump," I said, as I put her finger on my breast.

She said, "Wow, thanks so much. That was really helpful for me." I then told her I wanted to go home with a cane and asked when physical therapy was scheduled to come by. I was determined to keep the process moving forward, wanting to heal as quickly as I could so we could schedule the mastectomy.

Treatment Experience

In September 2014, I went in for my double mastectomy. I had decided on reconstructive surgery right afterward, so the surgeon put expanders in my breasts to hold the space in the muscle. She also removed five of my lymph nodes from my right breast that all tested negative. The doctor came by my room after the surgery and shared the news that she got good margins and didn't see any signs of cancer in my lymph nodes. I was free to move forward with my reconstruction, unless I wanted to go through chemotherapy and radiation treatment. I looked at her and shouted, "Hell no! I don't want to lose my hair." I was thirty-eight years old and loved my long hair. She smiled and talked about what would happen next. She gave me a prescription for Tamoxifen, a drug that was intended to prevent any chance of recurrence.

When I was moved from recovery to a hospital room, I learned that the hospital didn't have room on the oncology floor, so I was admitted to a room on a different floor. When I woke up in the night and had to go to the bathroom, I rang for a nurse to help me. She came into my room and said, "How do you want to get up? I am eight months pregnant. You are not putting me in labor tonight." *Wow, here I am the patient and recovering from major surgery, and she doesn't know what to do, how to help me to the bathroom. Really?*

She left and returned in a few minutes with the charge nurse, who said, "So how do you want us to do this?"

I was getting angry and shouted, "I don't know, I have never had this surgery before. I can't use my arms. Would you figure something out? I really have to go to the bathroom." They finally figured out to pull me up by my shoulders. I was ready to leave this hospital and regretted not having someone with me.

As I recovered, I found myself taking pain pills most days to be able to function normally with the expanders. They really hurt, like a deep muscle pain when you've been hit. The pain was frequent, although it occurred at random times and sometimes felt like muscle spasms all over my chest. I endured this process for several months before my reconstruction surgery. After my expansion process was over, I had to wait a couple weeks for my skin to calm down and was able to get my implants in January of 2015. Compared to my mastectomy, recovery from this procedure was minimal. I had drains for only a week and recovered quickly. I was delighted with the end result, although it was not a process I would have chosen.

A month later, I had my hands on my chest lying in bed watching TV and my pinky finger brushed over one of my scars on my right breast. I felt a lump in the exact same place as before! I thought, *Are you serious??* The next morning, I immediately called my breast surgeon and she fit me into her schedule later that day. She felt the lump and said she was pretty sure it was scar tissue but told me to call my oncologist and see what she recommended.

Hearing that my breast surgeon seemed so positive that it was only scar tissue gave me some relief. I went downstairs to my oncologist's office and asked if I could quickly talk to my doctor. She squeezed me into her packed schedule, and I was able to see her about thirty minutes later. She examined me and provided the same opinion as my breast surgeon—the lump was just scar tissue. Thankfully, she was a very cautious person and suggested I have another biopsy. I was able to get in for another biopsy the next day. As I drove to the appointment, I was calm. I had been through this procedure before and in my mind, I thought this procedure was no big deal because it was "just scar tissue."

A couple days later, my phone rang, and I noticed it was my oncologist. I was expecting to hear, *Yep, we were right. You're all good!* Sadly, that was not the case. My oncologist said, "Nikki, I'm really disappointed in your biopsy results." I was stunned beyond words. She continued, "It is unheard of for someone so young, on Tamoxifen, to get cancer back in less than four months." My ears started ringing, and I didn't hear much after that. I later found out my case was part of 2 percent of the population who do not respond to Tamoxifen. Unfortunately, the doctors were not able to know of my resistance to the drug until it didn't work. We hung up the phone after I confirmed another one of my fears, that this new discovery would require me to endure both chemotherapy and radiation. All through the process, I was angry and frustrated at times, although I was never afraid of the cancer. I believed that it wasn't going to beat me, because I had a son to live for. I was only afraid of the chemotherapy and radiation treatments and the impact each would have on my body.

Tuesday the following week, I went to a gynecological oncologist to see about getting a hysterectomy, due to testing positive for the BRCA2 gene. The doctor recommended a complete hysterectomy, which was a shock for me at just thirty-eight years old. The goal was to move fairly quickly, and my surgery was scheduled for later that week on Friday. Yes, another surgery. The previous year had been such a whirlwind of doctors and appointments and surgeries, I had a hard time keeping it all straight. The hysterectomy was performed laparoscopically, which led to a quicker recovery and minimal incisions. The downside was that the doctor pumped my body with air to be able to perform the procedure. I experienced an air bubble up under my collar bone, which felt like I was getting stabbed in the neck, off and on all day. I was grateful that bubble pain only lasted a week.

After I recovered, I went to see my breast surgeon. She planned to do a lumpectomy procedure in her office under local anesthesia, to save me money. My medical bills had mounted with all the surgeries I had endured. While this approach sounded good, it ended up being much more involved than either she or I thought. She found the first lump, and unfortunately then saw several more and continued cutting through a two-inch incision. After nineteen lidocaine injections, she decided to stop once she cut my chest wall. I flinched and almost catapulted off the table, as I felt it. She closed the incision and then looked at me and said, "Nikki, I am sorry. I was trying to save you money, and this didn't turn out like I thought. I would recommend you start chemotherapy infusions and let the medicine kill the cancer."

In March of 2015, I had healed enough to start Taxotere chemotherapy infusions. My dad went with me to every infusion and appointment. I was supposed to have six rounds, three weeks apart, and then have a Cytoxan infusion every third week. I started the Taxotere infusions and had an allergic reaction immediately, which my dad noticed, at the exact same time as Robyn, whose story is also in this book. The nurses swarmed to my side, stopped the infusion, gave me Benadryl and some steroids, and I started to feel better. It was a long eight-hour day, and I didn't get the full amount of medicine. The following week, my doctor recommended trying a different drug, Taxol. Within a few minutes, my throat started to close. I received the same Benadryl and steroids and didn't complete the infusion.

The next week, the doctor switched my medicine to Abraxane, which was a newer and more expensive drug. I endured fifteen weekly infusions. I experienced some nausea and felt extremely weak and tired, barely able to walk across the room some days or climb a few stairs. When I started losing my hair around my third week of treatment, I cut it very short. At the time, it stretched down to my lower back, and I wasn't quite ready to be bald yet. About a week later, my scalp started to ache. My husband had already shaved his head, so I asked him to shave mine. We went out to the garage, and he used the electric clippers and shaved off the rest of my hair. My seven-year-old son was so sweet and said he wanted to shave his head too. There we were, a family of baldies! I felt so supported, especially by my son being willing to join me in this experience.

At first, I was self-conscious about being a bald woman. I went to the cancer center's office and tried a wig to see what it would look like on me. I looked in the mirror and said, "No way, not for me!" It was not my style, and it felt uncomfortable. I thought about it and determined that there was enough I was going through—I didn't want to make myself more uncomfortable! I decided I had earned this bald head, and if it made someone else uncomfortable, that was their problem, not mine. If I needed to cover my head, I chose to wear a baseball cap. When it was too hot outside, I showed my bald head to the world.

I was so grateful to find people to bond with during chemotherapy. I still keep in touch with my group of chemotherapy friends, which we affectionately named the "Chemo Warriors." Now I pay it forward, staying in touch with those with whom I endured treatment and those now going through it. After my chemo infusions were finished, I had a PET scan to see how effective the treatment had been. I was told that there was no evidence of disease, although I didn't want to take any chances this time. I was given four weeks off before I started radiation. I endured thirty-five treatments, five days a week for seven weeks.

The radiation felt like a really, really deep sunburn, burning every cell in my body. I was grateful to have Jennifer's recommendation of using Aquaphor during the day, and Tamanu Oil at night. Once again, my dad took me to each appointment. There are no words to describe how loved and supported I felt by him, being with me every step of the way.

During my cancer treatment, I never asked myself why me, because I thought, *Why not me?* My dad had prostate cancer in 2014, and I went with him to chemotherapy infusions. In turn, he went with me to my infusions in 2015. Then he had to go back. We were battling together. During my treatment, I ended up gaining fifty pounds and had a really had a hard time losing the weight. When my treatment was complete, my doctor started me on Arimadex, which I will be on for another seven years.

I made a choice early on not to tell my seven-year-old son at the time that I had cancer, because I didn't want to scare him. I figured he wouldn't be shy about it and would tell people at school that his mom was sick. If he said I had cancer, they would likely tell him that he was going to lose his mom, which was not a risk I was willing to take. He knew I was sick, and I told him I would get better. After both of my surgeries, the hip and the double mastectomy, and when the cancer came back, I decided to tell my son that I was going to be very sick and would be bald soon. I shared that my hair would grow back after I was not sick anymore. I asked him if he had any questions about what was going on, as he knew I'd had hip surgery and surgery on my chest. My son looked at me and paused, scanning my body from my hip to my chest and said, "Why did they have to fix your hip by going through your boobs?" That struck me as so funny!

I laughed, looked at him, and said, "Honey I don't know, they do weird things for medical reasons." It brought some levity to a heavy conversation. When I finished my treatments and my hair started growing back, I was told that there was no evidence of disease. I decided then to tell my son that I'd had cancer, but there was nothing to worry about because I beat it. He is twelve now and knows about everything.

One of my greatest lessons in this whole experience is to trust my gut—if doctors are not doing what I think they should, I now push for answers and keep asking questions. As I reflect on this experience, I see how I learned to expect the unexpected at every turn. I am now grateful for each day I have. I believe everything happens for a reason, including people coming into my life. There is a reason. I now choose to be around the most positive people I can.

I tried to be so strong and did not let my husband know how hard it was as I was going through the cancer experience. He thought I didn't need anything as I showed a strong face to him. I wish I had been vulnerable and shared details with him, so he could have supported me better. It has been a valuable lesson for me to learn. While I grew up going to church, I used to only pray or talk to God when I needed something. This experience really changed me, and I now pray daily. My father lost his battle with cancer and died in September of 2016. My faith is what sustained me through that deep loss, as I was still recovering from so many surgeries.

Advice for Others

How I supported myself

- I did my best to keep a positive attitude and surrounded myself with the most positive people I could.
- I thanked God every day for waking up and having one more day.
- I laughed, smiled, and was an inspiration to others when the opportunity presented itself.
- I started praying daily and have continued this practice post-treatment.

How others supported me
- My dad took me to every appointment he could.
- I spent time with positive people.
- I relied on family and friends to support me.

Helpful tips
- If you are facing a diagnosis, I would recommend being vulnerable and sharing the details, so your spouse can support you; I wish I had done so.
- Be around the most positive people you can and focus on the good as much as possible.
- Be grateful for the day you have and make the most of it.
- Follow your gut—if doctors are not doing what you think they should, keep pushing for answers and keep asking questions.
- Expect the unexpected.

KIM'S STORY

———•━━●━━•———

I first started noticing some pressure in my throat in January of 2014. I had a regular practice of stretching about two to three times a week. One of the regular stretches I did while lying on the floor was to bring my legs over my head, then stretch my toes toward the floor. Increasingly over time, I felt more and more pressure in my neck and throat, but I had no other symptoms. I was reminded of this pressure only when I did this stretch. I started getting more curious about what this pressure might be and began noticing that when I gently touched the hollow notch in my neck, it was very sensitive to the touch, and I felt a slight gagging sensation. *Well that is weird, I'm not sure why that area is sensitive,* I thought. I started to research online and thought it might be a thyroid issue, although I wasn't having any other symptoms. In July, after this continued, I said to my husband, "I felt something strange in my throat when I was stretching this morning."

He replied, "I think you should get it checked out. Go to the doctor." I thought about it and brushed off his comment in my effort to minimize it. In late November, I started feeling achiness, pressure, and muscle fatigue in my neck. I shared it with my husband and once again, he said I should go to the doctor. I told him I would go after the holidays. Then the busyness of holiday preparations and gatherings of family and friends between Thanksgiving and Christmas took much of my time and attention. I started to feel more and more discomfort in my neck, and my throat was irritated from trying to swallow. I could no longer ignore it, and I knew that I would make an appointment as soon as the doctor's office was open after Christmas.

I am a nurse and worked ten to twenty hours a week as a patient advocate for a private client, which provided me a flexible schedule. Each morning, I tended to the important things I needed to do to keep strong spiritually, physically, and emotionally. I read my Bible, meditated on scripture passages, shared the concerns of my heart with Jesus, and took time to be still and quiet before God, so I could hear what God wanted to share with me. I loved to listen to music with words of life, and I often had it playing throughout the house. My daily routine included exercise and often a walk or hike with a friend. I loved being outside, especially with someone I enjoyed being with. Some days I would try to meet a friend in town for coffee before I headed to work for the afternoon. One day before Christmas, I was with a client and mentioned that I was having a hard time swallowing. She said, "Yes, Kim, it does seem to take you more effort to swallow. I've noticed that." I really didn't think anyone else could tell and was surprised that she noticed it.

After Christmas, I realized how tired I was and that my neck was really achy; if I wasn't looking straight ahead, my neck would get very tired. When I looked in the mirror, my neck appeared enlarged, and I noticed I didn't have the notch anymore. I realized this was not going away and was more than just being tired and rundown. I called the doctor and made an appointment. It was the day after Christmas, and I was able to schedule the appointment for New Year's Eve morning, which was a Wednesday. At this point, I knew something might be wrong. *Could this be cancer?* I wondered. I had minimized my symptoms to my husband and went to the appointment by myself. My doctor examined me as I talked through my symptoms. She said, "Kim, your thyroid feels enlarged. You will need an ultrasound so we can see what is going on. Let's schedule it as soon as possible." *Oh, okay, that's what it is.* I didn't want to jump to conclusions. *Or could this be cancer of the thyroid?* My mind starting racing forward, and I stopped it, refusing to jump ahead and go down the path of believing it was cancer. It was a pristine snowy day, and the air was crisp, perfect weather for a hike. When I arrived home, my husband and I prepared to go for a walk in the woods. While I was feeling rundown, I started to notice that I had the energy to do things once I was doing them. As we were walking to the trail head, my phone rang. It was the imaging center saying the ultrasound was set up for the following Monday at eleven, as the center was closed for the holiday. I hung up and told my husband, and we set out on our hike. Feeling the crisp air in my lungs help me relax and spending time in the trees with my husband filled my heart. I was excited about our New Year's Eve plans.

When we arrived back at our house, I noticed I had a missed call from my mom and there was a voice message. Before I had a chance to listen to it, my sister called and said, "Dad choked on a piece of steak during dinner. The ambulance is on its way."

Once I hung up with my sister, I called my mom. She said, "The paramedics came and are working on Dad and getting ready to transport him to the hospital. Please pray that they can help him. I feel so helpless and overwhelmed." I sat there staring at the phone, in shock and disbelief that this was really happening. When the paramedics got my dad in the ambulance, it took them a long time to remove the piece of steak, and my dad was without oxygen for over twenty minutes. I didn't know this until much later. My mom called me back when she was at the hospital, and I asked to talk to my dad. She put the phone up to his ear and I said, "Dad, I love you. Everything was going to be okay." He wasn't able to talk and was unresponsive, from what my mom said.

My dad was eighty-three years old and had stayed pretty healthy, going to the gym every day. He took a statin for high cholesterol. In the last year, I had started noticing that his muscular coordination was slowing down. He was more deliberate about using his arms, eating, and moving his legs, as if there was an issue with his nerve and muscle coordination. I closed my eyes and spoke to God, praying for grace and healing for my dad. I was hopeful that the doctors would be doing everything possible to revive him. I then noticed the time and remembered it was New Year's Eve. I told my husband I wanted to cancel our plans and be available to my mom if she called back. I just wanted to sit by the fire. My heart was breaking in two, and I was overwhelmed with grief. A waterfall of tears started pouring down my cheeks as I thought of my dad. I pondered how he was unresponsive and worried about if he did survive what kind of a life he would have. He didn't want to be kept alive on a machine. As I cried, it made everything worse in my head and neck.

I barely slept, tossing and turning, and woke up the next morning as my dad filled my thoughts. Suddenly my phone started ringing. It was my mother. She said, "Oh, Kim, I have some awful news. Your dad has died. It is my worst nightmare." She took a breath as I could hear her cry and sniffle. She continued, "I am trying to arrange for everyone to come into town so we can celebrate his life. He had decided to be cremated." I sat there in my bed still in shock from what she had said. I was wrestling with trying to find some comfort in the fact that my dad didn't suffer. A deep sadness started to permeate my body from my heart outward. Memories of my dad flooded my mind, knowing this was final and he was gone.

I took a deep breath, wanting to sound calm for her, and said, "Wow, just wow. I still can't believe what you just said. I saw a doctor yesterday about a lump in my throat, and I have an ultrasound scheduled for Monday." I took a breath and then continued, "I won't be able to come until at least next Friday."

She replied, "That's okay honey, you need to take care of yourself. It will give everyone time to schedule travel. We will do it next weekend. I love you." I told her I loved her, and we hung up.

My dad had just choked to death. As I sat there thinking of him and praying for my mom, memories of my grandfather, my dad's dad, filled my mind. Oh my goodness, he had also died from choking. He had been in a nursing home and died when they were feeding him, as he had pneumonia and was very weak. *Is choking that common? Seems like a crazy coincidence,* I thought. I was so devastated. I moved from my bed to the couch by the fire, still in my pajamas, feeling like my head was full of fog. I didn't move from that spot all weekend, and I don't remember eating. As my husband and friends tried to comfort me, I felt numb. I called my daughter and sons to let them know the terrible news. We were all in shock and so deeply sad.

Next thing I knew, it was Monday morning. I went to the ultrasound appointment by myself, as my husband was working. I will still in a zombie state as I lay down on the table. The technician looked over and asked, "How was your weekend?" as she put my information in the machine. I looked over at her and told her my dad had died, as tears started streaming down my face. She said she was so sorry in a very compassionate voice, and I felt comforted by her kind nature. As she moved the gel and wand over my throat, she said "Um, so this isn't just your thyroid. That's just the tip of it. I need to get the doctor to look at this. I'll be right back." She stepped out for a minute as the words permeated my foggy mind.

The radiologist came back with her, looked at the screen, and looked at me. He said, "We need you to have a CT scan with contrast soon; let's see what we can do to get you in this week." I was still in a daze about my father, and now it appeared something was more wrong than I'd thought. She tried to schedule the CT scan the same day but wasn't able to, likely due to the backup from the holiday. She came back and said it was set for Thursday morning.

I was still grieving deeply and just wanted to go home. I trusted God that the timing was right. I called my husband and told him about the ultrasound and that I had to have another test. When he got home, I shared more details, "This could be more and could be cancer. I am a little concerned."

When he realized it was more than my thyroid, he panicked. "This can't be happening!" he screamed. His fear took over, and he became anxious and angry as he continued, "How could this happen? How can it be?" I was watching him fall apart as both of us found it hard to believe. I have always been so healthy.

I replied, "Let's not go down that road yet. Let's take it one day at a time."

Besides my husband, I talked to my people—my mom, sister, children, friends, and neighbors—several times a day for the next few days. A few close friends came by and sat with me as well. I felt deeply supported, as if I were being carried by love and grace. I was still moving through my days surrounded by a grieving fog—I would start tending to a routine task and quickly forget what I was doing. I remember feeling, *When Thursday comes, I am going to have my scan and it will be okay, God is with me and going to help me through it.* I was at peace knowing, He was guiding the process. I could let go. Thursday came, and I went to the appointment. I went back for the scan feeling relaxed. It was very matter of fact, as they didn't have any results yet. The technician told me my doctor would call in a few days with the results. I went home to finish packing and focused on preparing to leave for several weeks, as our flight was scheduled for later in that afternoon.

While I was packing, my phone rang. I looked down and it was my primary care physician. *Wow that was fast*, I thought. I answered the phone and heard, "Kim, the scan showed some tumors in your chest, which could mean a couple of things. The first two possibilities are not cancerous but may require surgery. The third possibility is lymphoma, a blood cancer." I froze in my tracks as I processed what she had said. I had told her about my dad's death and asked her what I needed to do next, as I felt conflicted about wanting to stay behind and be with my mom for a while and needing to come back for appointments. I said, "Do you think it's okay for me to stay three weeks with my mom?"

She replied, "If it's any of these things, you are going to be okay when you come back. I believe you have enough time. This is what I think. I want you to see the thoracic surgeon and have the PET scan as soon as you come back to Colorado after visiting your mom. I think it will do your heart and soul good to spend time with her." She explained that waiting three weeks would be fine, although it was important to call this afternoon and get the appointments set for when I returned. I made a couple of calls and got both appointments scheduled for early February. With that behind me, I could shift back to where I was headed and the purpose of my trip, to celebrate my dad.

My mom and I enjoyed being together as we walked this path of deep grief and worked through Dad's affairs. We were still trying to process how his life ended so suddenly. Three weeks seemed to pass by quickly as we moved through our days in somewhat of a fog. On February 1, I flew home to Colorado and went with my husband to my appointment with the thoracic surgeon the next day. He recommended a thyroid biopsy in addition to the PET scan. We were in a holding pattern to learn more about what these tumors represented, so he explained what each test would show. I was still walking around in a fog, grieving, and the days came and went without much change. I had my PET scan on Friday, the sixth, and the biopsy the following Tuesday, the tenth. I had thought I would know something pretty quickly and called two or three times to follow up, only to hear that all the results were not back. I thought, *I have had this lump in my throat for over a year. I can wait a few more days.*

On February 23, 2015, my phone rang around eight at night, and it was my primary care physician. I paused as I answered, concerned that she was personally calling me so late in the day.

She said, "Kim, I have some news for you. The results showed you have non-Hodgkin's lymphoma, diffuse large B-cell. There were actually four tumors that showed up, the largest one was in your throat and was seven by five centimeters. The other three tumors are smaller." As the words permeated my mind, I thanked God for the large tumor. The smaller tumors would have gone on growing, unnoticed, if it hadn't been for the tumor in my throat. My doctor continued, in a compassionate voice, "There is aggressive cancer in your lymphatic system." She then explained the details of B-cells and T-cells and why it was considered an aggressive cancer. I sat there completely dumbfounded by what I was hearing. I started feeling sick to my stomach. She continued to explain the type of cancer and that I would need chemotherapy and radiation.

I asked, "Am I going to lose my hair? I love my hair."

She replied, "Yes, you probably will lose your hair. Kim, I want to leave this call with giving you hope, though. We have had good results with the treatment. I think you will be fine." Tears started streaming down my cheeks. I thanked her and hung up as I went looking for my husband. I shared the news with him, and we both fell apart, clinging to each other as we sorted out this news. I was more afraid of the prospect of the chemotherapy and other treatment than the cancer. We both cried and prayed together, and then we called each of our three children and told them. Each of my children was thoughtful and tried to comfort me and give me hope. The reality that I had cancer right after my dad had died was so devastating. We were already so swallowed up by sadness. I wondered, *How much can we handle at one time?* Everything was so overwhelming. The only thing holding me together was my relationship with Jesus.

Feeling somewhat lost and wanting to regain control, I reached out for referrals from friends the next day. I had two appointments, one the following Monday and one Tuesday. I also called the oncologist office that my primary care physician recommended and left a message. I was determined to explore several options and make sure I made the best choice to give me the highest chance of survival. My husband went with me the following Monday to the first appointment. As we interviewed the first oncologist, she did not convey confidence in her ability to treat me and seemed unsure of how she would proceed. She waited for me to ask questions and only then gave vague information. My husband asked a lot of questions about the treatment protocol for the specific type of cancer, and she vaguely answered him. I left that appointment feeling somewhat discouraged.

The next day I had an appointment with a naturopath. The treatment she proposed was for eight months, very expensive, and not covered by insurance. She used a lot of fear to try to convince me that the medical treatment would be harmful to me and was not in my best interest. Red flags came up for me as I did not feel like this doctor was a good choice for me. I continued to feel very lost and confused.

After the appointment with the second doctor on Tuesday, I knew that neither of these doctors was right for me. About an hour later, I got a call from the oncologist whom my primary care physician recommended. He wanted me to come in the following morning. I called my dear friend to tell her how my day was going, and she wanted to go with me for my appointment the next morning. That was comforting for me. Before I went to sleep that night, I asked God to give me help and guidance. That night, I had a dream that is still as vivid as it was in that moment. As I was walking across the street, a red car came barreling down the street, heading right for me. Realizing that I would be hit if I didn't get out of the way; I screamed and quickly jumped back and then woke up. I thought, *Hooray, I'm alive! I'm not dead.* I was exhausted. I prayed again, "God, if this message is from you, let me remember it in the morning. Will you remind me?" I took several deep breaths to calm me from the fear in the dream and was able to go back to sleep. My dream was the first thing I thought of when I woke up. I prayed and asked God to explain what the dream meant. I heard,

Aggressive attack, urgent response, which to me meant I needed to move forward quickly with treatment.

Later that morning, which was March 4, I went with my dear friend to interview the oncologist recommended by my primary care doctor. I knew he was the right doctor by his calm nature and the compassionate way he talked to me. He gave me so much hope. He explained everything with just the right amount of detail, whether I asked the right questions or not. He then said, "The lymphoma you have is aggressive; on a scale of one to ten, ten being the most aggressive, your diagnosis is an eight. We need to get on this ASAP." After explaining the details, he said in a caring voice, "Next you will need an echocardiogram, and have a port-a-cath installed. Your chemotherapy infusions will be every three weeks and can start after your port is installed. Be prepared to feel sick for one and a half to two weeks after the infusions." He also said that I needed to attend a class with my family and friends to learn more about the medical and practical information we needed to know for my treatment and care. I was able to get them all scheduled quickly.

Treatment Experience

I was able to have the bone marrow biopsy just two days later, on Friday, March 6. It was a very uncomfortable test. I had the echocardiogram the following Monday, March 9, and went into surgery on Wednesday, March 11, to install the port-a-cath. The procedure to insert the port was in the operating room under sedation. While I thought the bone marrow test was uncomfortable, recovering from this surgery was tougher than any other part of the preparation. I went to the pre-treatment class on Friday, March 13, with the infusion nurse, my son, and seventeen friends who came to support me. I was very touched as I looked around the room. My chemotherapy regimen was known as R-Chop. I received infusions every three weeks, with a PET scan after the first two rounds and again after the fourth round to determine how the cancer was responding. Depending on the results of the PET scan, I would endure four or six infusions. After chemotherapy, I was scheduled for twenty radiation treatments, one a day, Monday through Friday, for four weeks.

On March 16, 2015, I started my chemotherapy infusions. My husband brought me and stayed with me all day. I was required to bring all the medication and supplements I was taking to this first appointment, along with food, my pillow, blanket, and anything else I wanted. When my doctor came into the room, he joked and said, "This is ridiculous, are you going to move in?" which made me laugh and lightened my mood for something that I was apprehensive about. I was taking a lot of supplements at the time, and the doctor went through each one and told me which ones I needed to stop. I needed to discontinue anything processed through my liver, such as roots like turmeric. The drug regimen was a really harsh medicine that would take a huge toll on my liver. I was grateful that the doctor was willing to work with me and let me keep taking some supplements. He then said, "I believe you are going to wipe out the cancer and live a long life." He gave me hope, and I believed him.

As I scanned the room, taking in my new surroundings and preparing for my first infusion, I said under my breath, *Okay God, if this is why I am here, show me who I need to pray for.* I walked by a man who was wearing leather chaps and a bandana to get to my infusion chair as he said, "Hi, beautiful." I affectionately named him the "Harley guy." It made me smile and calmed my nerves. As the infusion began, I became very sleepy. A very sweet couple came to visit me, and they prayed for me. After they left, I wanted to make the most of my circumstances.

I heard in my spirit, *You need to pray for him*, meaning the Harley guy. I was mentally, physically, and emotionally drained of energy. Although I knew praying was important, I was struggling to gather my thoughts. He walked past me, and I whispered, "I need to pray for you."

He smiled and went to the bathroom. When he came back, he whispered, "I need to pray for you, too."

I was pleasantly surprised and said, "Okay," under my breath. I felt my energy shift to a lighter feeling, and my fuzzy mind became clear right after that. I needed clarity in order to pray for him. After we prayed for one another, we kept in touch and tried to encourage each other and the other people we met during infusions.

After my first infusion, I felt pretty woozy and disoriented when I got home from the hospital. I didn't realize that what I was feeling were the signs that I should take anti-nausea medication, because it wasn't exactly nausea. But as more time went on, I did feel nauseous and at that point it, the anti-nausea medication wasn't very effective. I felt nauseous all night, but I did not vomit, which I was so thankful for. My husband took me to the hospital the next day to get IV fluids and the injection to activate my bone marrow to increase the production of blood cells that would replace those that were being destroyed by the chemotherapy drugs. A few days later, my mom flew into Colorado from Pennsylvania to help me.

When we went to my one-week follow-up visit, the doctor said, "Remember, Kim, you should expect to lose your hair around twenty-one days after your first infusion." *Wow, and there it is. I am going to lose the hair I so love.* I was so grateful to have my mom with me as I processed my new reality, the most physical sign that I was a cancer patient. I told him I was very nauseous after the first round, and he said he would add more anti-nausea meds to the chemo to help with that. I also told him that I had been extremely weak at times, often feeling like I was going to pass out. My legs felt like they were going to buckle under me, and my blood sugar and blood pressure seemed really low. He believed these symptoms were caused by adrenal fatigue, so after each round he would wean me off the prednisone gradually instead of just stopping it five days after the infusion. I felt supported by him and listened to, validating my choice of doctors and my willingness to speak up about how I was feeling. Before we left the cancer center, my mom and I picked out a free wig. On the way back home, we stopped and bought a couple of fun hats. Two friends let me use their wigs, which I so appreciated. I also started collecting scarves to wrap around my head when I didn't feel like wearing a wig or a hat.

The day before Easter, April 4, my hair was falling out in clumps and handfuls, about the time the doctor said it would. I decided it was time to shave my head. My husband offered to shave it while my mom and two of our children watched. I felt deeply supported, and they made me laugh, as they said I had a beautifully shaped head! I sent a picture to my dear friend who had come to my doctor's appointment with me. A couple hours later, she sent me a picture of her bald head, and I cried, overwhelmed with gratitude by her choice to do that in support of me. I would never ask or expect anyone to do that! The following day, we invited our son, his wife, and her family over for Easter dinner, and everyone pitched in to help with the meal preparation. I revealed my bald head again, which shocked everyone who hadn't yet seen me. The expression on my middle son's face was priceless. The day after Easter, my husband brought me, my mom, and my daughter to the hospital for my second round. Friends came to see me and meet my mom and daughter, who were staying with me. At the end of the day, a friend came to bring the three of us home. I felt less nauseous this time, although constipation was a new side effect that was not easy to manage. Following the second infusion, the PET scan showed that the tumors were shrinking nicely, which gave me hope and energy to keep fighting.

For my third infusion, my neighbor and dear friend, who had gone through the same cancer, brought me to the hospital, and another dear neighbor brought me back home at the end of the day. Friends and neighbors visited me, read to me (my eyes were so dry and my vision so blurry that I couldn't read), and dropped off smoothies and meals regularly. I was well cared for and felt loved. I would always have enough energy to visit, as it encouraged me, but right after anyone left, I felt very tired and usually slept. I listened to a lot of uplifting music, and when I felt strong enough, I would go for a walk. I sat outside on my deck as much as I was able. A week after my third infusion, my husband wanted to climb the incline in Manitou Springs, Colorado. I decided to go with him and just do what I felt comfortable doing. I climbed very slowly and told him to go on ahead. Along the way, I met several people who encouraged me and to my great surprise, I got all the way to the top and then hiked down on Barr Trail. My heart expanded as I breathed in the mountain air and felt strong and somewhat normal, putting out of my mind that I was a cancer patient.

My sister flew in from Ohio to be with me for my fourth infusion. She met some of the friends who came to visit and also several of the patients I had gotten to know. My sister stayed with me for two weeks, and we had a great time together. We spent time every morning sharing what we were learning and loving about Jesus. She and my daughter-in-law helped me plan our daughter's wedding shower, and my family stepped in to help in such a big way on the day we pulled it all together. After the fourth infusion, the PET scan showed that the tumors were gone, and I could start radiation. It was just the right time as the chemotherapy regimen was taking more and more out of me with each infusion, and I didn't think I would make it through two more rounds. I was getting weaker, and it was getting more difficult to speak and project my voice.

I had to be measured and tattooed before I began radiation to make sure that I was radiated in the exact same place each time. I started radiation in mid-June. My skin did burn a bit, but I kept it moisturized, and it never got too bad. I got a massage once a week to help with the muscle tightness that was a side effect of the radiation. I also temporarily lost my voice as it affected my vocal chords. Each day when I climbed up on the radiation table,

I would remember to surrender my life for the purposes that God had created me for. I was trusting God for complete healing, but I also trusted that He had good plans for me whether or not I was healed, and I was at peace with that. On the last day of my twenty radiation treatments over four weeks, a very dear friend picked me up at my house, brought me to the hospital, took me to lunch to celebrate the last day, and then brought me back home. She went way out of her way, so I didn't have to drive at all. I was very touched by the generous love she showed me.

One memorable experience during treatment was a luncheon that the Harley rider I met at the cancer center told me about. I hadn't officially met the woman hosting it yet, but I wanted to go, even though it was an hour away from my house. I felt in my soul it was important that I go. I picked up some flowers and drove the hour to her house, rang the doorbell, and waited for someone to let me in. She opened the door and I said, "Do you know the Harley rider? I'm looking for a luncheon with ladies who have been through cancer treatment. I think I found you since we all have the same hairstyle! He told me about the luncheon today, and I brought these flowers for you!"

She said yes, she knew him and welcomed me in. There were three other ladies, who each share their stories in another chapter of this book: Robyn, Nikki, and Jennifer. The five of us sat around the table and shared stories, getting to know each other. I asked each one if I could pray for them individually during the afternoon, and they gave me the wonderful opportunity to do that. Our friend who had told me about the luncheon dropped by, and we took pictures, shared more stories, and prayed for him as well. We began a support group and called ourselves the "Chemo Warriors." Many others joined us, and we met once a month until many of us started moving out of the area. We supported each other through many storms. To this day, we still text each other and lift each other up. No one should go through trials and hardship alone; we all need people in our lives who care.

Before my cancer diagnosis, I was pretty strong willed and independent, not really wanting to rely on anyone. With all the appointments and treatments, I learned to open up more and let others who cared about me help. Some things were hard for me to hear as I navigated the unknown waters of cancer treatment. I always want people to be honest, but sometimes people can be too honest or say things that don't need to be said. There were times I felt like a burden to my husband, children, extended family, and friends as the circumstances surrounding cancer and treatment got in the way of what I—and we—wanted life to look like. Cancer really opened up my spiritual eyes to see what was going on in me— my fears, insecurities, sensitivities, and anxious thoughts and how they impacted the way I related to others. We all want to be in control, and when we aren't, we can get angry and behave in ways that reveal or reflect our inner world. My husband and I had some heart-to-heart conversations and decided to get help to better understand each other and learn better ways to communicate. We continue to work on this, for which I am thankful.

Another thing I had to change as a result of being diagnosed with cancer was finding my voice. I am a pretty easygoing person, and I would speak up when things really mattered to me. Many times, I had been comfortable going along with what my husband, family, or friends wanted, but if I felt strong enough to speak up about something, I wanted to be acknowledged. There were often times when I felt my voice was not valued, and I just deferred to someone else. I suspect that I might have lost my sense of self along the way. When I was going through treatment, I became very aware that it was important to speak up for myself because no one could possibly know how I felt or what I needed. Entertaining was not something I had the energy for. I learned to speak up to address my needs, and I tried to do it graciously, but there were times when others got hurt, and I just had to let it go.

Through this journey, I have become more aware of stress and how it impacts me and my body. I hold a lot of stress in my neck and shoulders, and I knew this could really impact the health of my lymphatic system in this area. As a result, I am now more committed to making decisions that promote relaxation and rest and provide time to do the things that bring me a feeling of zest and enjoyment. I love to spend time meditating on the fullness of life with Jesus using practical tools. I now prioritize time to do this and to spend time with people who are wise and life giving. The Bible is full of truth and wisdom, and I believe it is vital for me to study it in order to have an anchor for my life. I have added a rich practice of gratitude and thankfulness that has brought me so much joy. I also have prioritized time to have fun, laugh, and do things I love. I have learned the importance of taking time to be filled with the rich life that only our creator, God, can give, and when I am full, I have enough love and light to share with others. I am thankful that the cancer experience taught me to live more intentionally in the present.

Advice for Others

How I supported myself
- Prayed throughout the day, sharing my heart with God and listening for His words and requests for me.
- Read the Bible.
- Took time for myself, spent time outside in nature.
- Spent time with life-giving, truth-telling, loving people.

How others supported me
- My husband, family, and friends supported me through every step of the treatment.
- Friends and family members brought meals, CDs, DVDs, and smoothies and drove me to places I wanted to go or appointments I needed to attend.
- Friends ran errands for me, like picking up groceries, medications, or anything else I needed.
- Friends and family members sent me cards and flowers.

Helpful tips

- Know that the person who has cancer is navigating life from a whole new perspective, learning new things about their body and the treatment every day; it can be exhausting to also entertain loved ones and friends.
- Know that cancer patients want to be engaged with life and people, so engage and don't avoid them, although they may need to take visits in smaller doses; they need encouragement and hope, so be generous with love!

GINA'S STORY

———•—●—•———

I was thirty-four in October of 2001 and adjusting to life with a two-year-old. I was an extensive breastfeeding mom, still supplementing my daughter's meals with the comforts and nourishment of breast milk. One day as I was breastfeeding her, I noticed a lump on my left breast. As I rubbed my finger over it, I jumped a little as it was painful to touch and felt like a knot. I had experienced a plugged milk duct before and thought it was likely an intense duct issue, but when the lump size did not reduce even after warm compressions, I went to my nurse midwife. She examined me and diagnosed it as a bad case of mastitis with reassurance that my worse-case-scenario thoughts of cancer were not part of her assessment; in her experience, cancer does not hurt, but mastitis can be very painful. She prescribed antibiotics, and I expected the lump would go away.

Between running a company and raising a two-year-old, life was crazy and all of a sudden it was February of 2002. The lump was still there, and my daughter was not interested in feeding off that breast. I went back to my nurse midwife. Again, she examined me and said it was nothing to worry about, that mastitis can be difficult. I insisted that something more must be wrong—I had taken the medicine, used warm compressions, and the lump seemed to be larger, harder, and more painful. After looking over my chart, she scheduled a mammogram on my birthday, because my insurance would pay for it once I turned thirty-five years old.

The night before the mammogram, I shared my deep concerns and fear with my husband, with our conversation ending on a positive note that all would be okay. With butterflies in my stomach, I drove myself to my very first mammogram and arrived early on my birthday appointment. I was called back pretty quickly, and as the technician started the mammogram, she asked if it was a diagnostic mammogram. I replied, "No, this is my first screening mammogram." After several positions and images, the technician left the room for a minute, saying she would be right back. She returned with the radiologist, who explained that something had shown up and asked if I had time to wait for a diagnostic ultrasound.

I waited and waited as fear and anxiety started to build inside my body, making it challenging to focus on a story in the magazine I was flipping through. I finally pulled out my cell phone and called my sister, asking her to make arrangements for our children to be picked up from daycare and to come join me at the hospital. I kept replaying the conversation and the look on the technician's face in my mind, and I knew in my heart that the "nothing" lump would be something serious. I imagined I would need her support, her ears to listen with me when the doctor spoke, a shoulder to cry on, and a fresh brain not clouded by hours of waiting and months of concern. After over two hours, I was finally called back. A technician started the ultrasound, measuring spots that I could see on the screen, all the while looking at me and back at the screen.

By the time my sister arrived, the technician had left to find the radiologist. When she came back in, the radiologist was looking over the images and pointing to a mass, which looked the size of a grapefruit. It was rounded from the front and resembled a cluster of grapes on the sides. Even though I was expecting bad news, I was still in shock as I stared at the screen, remembering the past six months and the times my nurse midwife had told me it was nothing more than plugged duct or mastitis. The radiologist looked at me with grave concern and said, "Gina, this is pretty serious. I recommend you make an appointment with a breast surgeon before you leave here today." I asked several times for an explanation of the mass and received the same reply, "You need a biopsy with a breast surgeon." No one said the word "cancer," but I was not in the dark about what the technician and radiologist were implying in their words of grave concern.

I thanked her and explained that we were leaving early in the morning for our first family Disney World vacation and would be gone for ten days. She reiterated her concerns and gave me prescriptions for anxiety and sleep medicines. With the prescriptions in my hand, I went to leave, feeling strongly that cancer was the likely outcome. I promptly scheduled the appointment for the day after we returned.

I went home and told my husband about the spot that was found, the concerned radiologist, and my appointment with a breast surgeon upon our return. I purposely did not describe just how serious it might be. Just eighteen months earlier, my dad had died of lung cancer, and after walking the path with him, I knew we could be facing months of treatment and fear. In discussion with my husband, I insisted that we keep our vacation plans. I knew in the back of my mind that it would be a while before we could travel again, and there was a realistic possibility that this could be our first and last family vacation. It was not easy, but necessary to ignore my fear and focus on enjoying my sweet family on this magical adventure. I was grateful to have medicine from the radiologist to ease anxiety and aid in my ability to sleep, although I didn't use either one. Knowing I had the medication was comforting and enabled me to maintain a calm demeanor and sleep soundly. Based on what I experienced with my dad's cancer journey and given what I understood about my own health situation, I chose to treasure every memory and take in each moment, one at a time, not knowing what would happen when we returned.

Upon returning from our magical Orlando vacation, reality set in with an eerie silence in the air and the weight of the impending biopsy, as I moved around like a robot and felt numb. I arranged for my sister and mother to meet my husband and me at the surgical oncology office. My husband and I were called back while my sister and mother sat holding hands in the waiting room. My ultrasound images had been sent to the doctor from the hospital, and we were told that a core biopsy was scheduled. I was given a local anesthetic, and while we waited for the numbing to take effect, my husband and I studied the charts and posters on the walls in our room, which explained different breast abnormalities including cancer. After seeing these images, in my heart and mind, I was preparing myself for the worst possible outcome.

During the procedure, the doctor and nurses calmly talked us through each step, asking if I was feeling any pain, while explaining why a core biopsy was necessary. When the procedure was complete, the doctor focused on my husband and me and said the words I had been dreading: "Until we have the pathology lab work, it is not confirmed, but in my professional experience, this is a malignant mass or tumor." My husband was speechless as tears streamed down my face.

I had to ask, "Are you sure?"

He replied, "Yes, unfortunately so. The lab work will confirm in a few days." The doctor explained that speaking to an oncologist was my next step to form a plan of action and then continued to describe briefly what the different types of surgery might be, from lumpectomy, mastectomy, to bilateral mastectomy, as we pelted him with questions. I had my first crash course on breast cancer terminology and procedures that day. When the doctor and nurse left the room, I hugged my husband so tight, not wanting to let go, and broke down into uncontrollable tears. The first bomb of this cancer war had dropped, and I felt the weight of the world on me. I assumed I was dying, as that is what had happened to my dad. I wondered what would become of my daughter.

When the nurse reappeared to check on us, I asked if she could send my mother and sister to our room. We all cried as we hugged each other, still in shock at how quickly our lives had changed. It seemed like we were there for hours and maybe we were—time seemed to stop, allowing us to absorb the devastating news. When we emerged from the room, the nurse said that they had made an appointment for me with an oncologist for the following week. I would learn the results of the test at that appointment. The procedure had not been painful, although I was told that mild to significant discomfort and bruising would follow, which is what I experienced.

I was able to shift my focus to taking care of my daughter and running my business, distracting me in a helpful way from my new reality. The week went by faster than I expected. When my husband, sister, and I arrived at the oncologist's office, I was pleasantly surprised to find it nicely decorated and comforting, which was different than my experience with my dad's doctors. I noticed that my oncologist was actually a hematologist-oncologist, which somehow gave me extra comfort and confidence, a feeling that he was well qualified. The nurse called me back, weighed me, took my blood pressure and temperature, and then drew several blood samples. I experienced my first vasovagal syncope as the nurse drew blood—my heart rate and blood pressure plummeted, and the next thing I remember, I was being transferred into a wheelchair. I had been present for my dad's blood draws with no issues, so I had no idea that I would faint. It's possible that my fainting was related to the emotional distress I was feeling over the situation. I was advised to ask to lie down before my next blood draw, which I happily agreed to.

The doctor came in and introduced himself then shared my results. He said, "Gina, the results came back. You do have a malignant tumor, called HER2/neu, over expressive three plus and negative in hormones, estrogen and progesterone." He shifted to explain what would happen next—a CT scan, followed by chemotherapy, surgery, and radiation. We were all focused on his words and his description of what HER2/neu meant. At the time and from what I understood, only 15 percent of breast cancers turned out to be HER2/neu, which is considered very aggressive in growth, typically found in younger patients. He told us that some cutting-edge drugs, which targeted HER2 proteins, were possibly available. He had a matter-of-fact way of giving the information while he remained very positive that we would have a treatment plan soon. We would know more once we had the CT scan results. Before I left his office, my CT scan was scheduled as well as a return visit within the same week. The three of us left with our current questions answered but unsatisfied because so many more questions were looming. I felt numb and detached, as if this was someone else's story.

My sister volunteered to pick up our two-year-old daughter after school indefinitely, as she knew we were uncertain of our constantly changing daily schedule. Two days later, my husband and I arrived for my first of several CT scans. The technician was very kind to explain the procedure. My CT scan was ordered with contrast, which is a type of dye that emphasizes certain features, and during the injection process causes the patient to feel the need to pee. And it *did*! My fear turned to discomfort as I thought I might pee on myself on this cold, sterile, narrow, stainless steel table in what felt like a freezing room. The nurse saw me shivering and quickly brought me a blanket. Surrounded by compassionate nurses and technicians, I was humbled by their ability to do their job with kindness. I thought about how they must see many patients with life-threatening diagnoses who are anxious and difficult. That day, I made a goal to be the best patient I could be, as this diagnosis was nobody's fault—not mine, not my family's, friends', caregivers', or doctors', and ultimately, we would become a team of cancer fighters, together.

When I arrived home, I called a dear friend and business colleague in New York City. His mother had just experienced cancer treatments at one of the top ten cancer centers, and within minutes, I scheduled an appointment a week later for a second opinion. On my return visit to the first oncologist I saw, I was accompanied by my posse—my husband, sister, dearest childhood friend, and my older brother from my father's previous marriage, who fortunately was a pathologist-toxicologist and well versed in all things we were about to discuss. The oncologist dropped the second bomb of my cancer battle. He said, "Gina, not only is your cancer a rare HER2/neu over-expressive, hormone negative, and aggressive, the CT showed it is a five-by-eight-centimeter mass about equal to a small grapefruit or a large orange. We saw another mass on your kidney and several questionable spots in your liver. These findings change your diagnosis to a stage III B." I sat there dumbfounded by this news, not able to find any words. Given my cancer diagnosis, my oncologist proposed a study by a local female doctor who was researching HER2/neu—with a special cocktail of experimental drugs. We thanked him and went home, and then started preparing for my New York appointment. I was still in shock from the new discovery and continued in my robotic way of moving through my days.

The following week came quickly, and we arrived at the appointment in New York. The doctor introduced herself, examined me, and looked over my scans and pathology results. She looked at me and said, "Gina, here is what I would recommend: start with a breast MRI for detailed imaging of the tumor, next have a sentinel node biopsy with mastectomy to remove the tumor in your body, and then enter a clinical drug trial." She continued explaining more about the drug trial—the downside of the trial was that only half of the patients would receive the drug Herceptin (HER2/neu-targeted drug) and the other half received a placebo in place of Herceptin. As I processed these words, I connected the dots that choosing this option meant there was a fifty-fifty chance I would not receive any drugs during the trial, allowing the cancer to continue to spread without treatment. She shared that the breast

MRI was a new innovation and only available in a couple of locations. I took it all in, still in my detached state. At every meeting, I learned new terminology and got information about another drug or procedure option.

After leaving New York, we immediately drove to Little Rock, Arkansas, where the breast MRI had been invented by a local doctor. Fortunately for me, my older brother lived there, and we were able to stay in his loving home, making our stay more comfortable. At that time, this new technology was not covered by insurance and cost over $12,000 out of pocket each visit. We agreed to the test, as this new technology was really important to me to understand the full scope of the cancer and visualize its mass. The scan was revealing and confirmed calcifications in my left breast. I left thinking we would likely be back for a second scan at an approximate total cost of $25,000.

My next appointment was back in Nashville with my surgical oncologist. After learning about the sentinel node biopsy, I explained to my surgeon that I wanted him to perform the surgery and install a port-a-cath for chemotherapy at the same time, allowing me to only go under anesthesia once. He said that was an unusual request, but he agreed to do it. I requested the port because I watched my father struggle through chemotherapy, as his veins were difficult to find. I was determined to have a different experience. The sentinel node surgery included a shot of dye that followed the cancer to the furthest node affected, resulting in further understanding of the cancer.

The next day was my decision appointment with my local oncologist. Before that appointment, I decided I wanted yet another opinion and reached out to one more well-known cancer treatment center with my diagnosis, pathology, and scan information. I was given similar recommendations to the plan offered in New York. My thought process in getting the second and third opinions revolved around my being fully on board with the treatment offered by my doctor, whichever one I chose. I knew instinctively, once I made a decision, I would be able to concentrate on surviving. For me, knowledge was power, and with this knowledge, I would face the cancer with strong armor. Seeking knowledge from multiple reputable sources helped give me peace that I had turned over every stone and had all the information to make an informed decision. At the time of my diagnosis, 85 percent of breast cancer patients were being diagnosed with the same type of cancer, and they would receive the same drug regimen. With my two-year-old on my mind constantly, I pushed the boundaries and looked for any new procedure or drugs that might increase my chances of survival.

The next day, we arrived with much more information and many new questions. My oncologist explained the special cocktail drug trial he offered, which did not included Herceptin. He explained that Herceptin was only offered in drug trials, and while only 50 percent of patients would receive the drug, in his experience, if Herceptin was successful in that drug trial, we would have access to Herceptin if I needed it for future treatments in the event that the cancer returned. Then I asked an emotionally charged question: "I would like to know what my chances of surviving are. I have a two-year-old and run a family business that includes traveling every month. I also manage my father's trust for my mother. I need to know the truth in order to prepare adequately while I am still feeling well." When my father was fighting cancer, his clinical team seemed to dance around the subject of death, not addressing the topic in a straightforward manner, and it felt like no one had a sense of urgency.

My doctor replied, "We will give it eighteen months, and if your body responds well to treatment, we will plan for three years. If the cancer comes back at a later date, we will have Herceptin as a backup plan." Given my Eastern medicine upbringing, I truly believed that no one would be able to predict the exact outcome. Upon hearing these short time frames, I gulped so loud it was probably heard down the hall. I took a deep breath and set my mind on fighting this cancer battle with every possible resource while I realistically planned for the worst.

Once I believed in my treatment and my doctor, I knew instinctively that I would be able to concentrate better and focus on healing my body and facing the cancer with strong armor. Once my family knew about my health situation, I had told them to ask whatever questions they wanted, and that there were no stupid questions. And so they did, through the whole process. We were a team, and I believed what we did not understand, we feared. We learned together as I fielded questions and found answers.

Treatment Experience

My first step in the treatment process was a sentinel node biopsy and installation of a port-a-cath. Next I would endure chemotherapy infusions, have surgery, endure more chemotherapy, and possibly have radiation. I wanted to have chemotherapy before the surgery so I would know whether the chemo was shrinking the tumor. My spiritual upbringing was a mixture of cultures and beliefs. My Japanese mother's Buddhist Eastern approach included meditation and chanting while focusing on positive energy rolling through my body. My father was Jewish and had his own beliefs. And my husband and I attended Christian chapel Sunday services at my daughter's school. I was determined to do all I could to survive. I prayed daily and spoke to the cancer, saying "You are dying. I'm giving you poison. You are going away, shrinking, and soon we are cutting you out. You are going *down*—get *out*!"

I was surrounded by love and support from my family and friends during my treatment. One special memory is when my younger brother came to town before my first chemotherapy infusion. He said to me, "You were the first to be born, first to graduate high school, first to get married, and first to have babies. You are *not* going to be first to lose your hair." We were standing in the kitchen at the time. He left and came back with a razor, and then my baby sister shaved his head in front of me and my daughter. I felt humbled and surrounded by love. His goal was to make shaving my head not scary for my daughter, as I had heard of another story of a mom coming home with a shaved head and her young child running away, screaming, "*Monster!*" A week later, when I went to have my head shaved, I took my daughter with me. When my head was shaved, she looked at me and said, "You look just like your brother!" I was so grateful that my brother had shaved his head, as it made my bald head look normal in my daughter's eyes. It may sound silly, but losing my hair tore me apart inside and was the first visible sign that I was a cancer patient. I'd had long hair almost to my waist, and losing it reinforced my new reality.

My chemotherapy drug regimen consisted of the following drugs: Rubix and Doxil, known as Red Devil, Taxotere, and Gemzar. These medicines were considered very strong and would possibly put undue stress on my heart. In addition to a PET scan, I had a baseline cardiac test before starting chemotherapy. Gemzar was a pancreatic cancer drug, which was demonstrating positive results with HER2/neu proteins. I started the infusions in late June and had Red Devil and Taxotere on Thursdays and, the following Thursday, I had infusions with Gemzar, and then took one week off before beginning the next round. During the treatments, I felt extremely tired and weak, as if my muscles had atrophied. By mid-August after my third round, my blood counts were extremely low, leading me to have a blood transfusion. I lacked the energy to walk upstairs to my daughter's bedroom, so my husband moved her downstairs to be with us. I endured eight rounds of the two-week drug regimen, and then took eight weeks for my body to recover before my surgery.

My husband is typically the eternal optimist, although my cancer diagnosis changed that. I could see he was very scared. I gave him lists of things to do and people to call to keep him focused on something else. I remained positive and armed for battle to fight for survival, while preparing for the worst, as I did not want to leave a burden behind for anyone if the treatment failed. I wrote down details so my husband would know how to run the house alone, including a grocery list of all the things we ate, especially our daughter's favorites, in the form of a checklist. I made a list of house chores that I carried out weekly, monthly, and annually. I created folders with letters of "what to do in case" checklists for my office and my trust attorney. My husband took me to every appointment except for one or two. Sometimes he would lie on the floor in the bathroom in the middle of the night with me while I curled in a fetal position, crying in severe pain. I could tell by the look on his face that I looked like death. He asked. "Do you need to go to the ER?" I told him they would not be able to do anything to help me, it was just part of the treatment process.

My mother is a nurturer and derives joy from serving others. She would cut up raw veggies and fruit to juice and would bring them to me during each infusion. The combination of juicing and Reiki (stress reducing and relaxation technique from Japan) was her Eastern medicine approach to help me heal. Knowing the chemotherapy caused extreme dehydration, I drank eight bottles of water a day; I marked the bottles "one" through "eight" to ensure I didn't miss one.

After my fourth round of chemotherapy, I had my second blood transfusion, as I was extremely weak and limp like a ragdoll. I felt literally like I was dying and that things could not get worse. I accepted what I felt was God's plan, inviting death in and acknowledging that I was at peace if it was my time. I felt liberated and well prepared, with checklists and letters to my loved ones, along with designated successors. I felt God's presence with me from the very beginning of my diagnosis. Growing up in a small town, my siblings and I had an eclectic religious and spiritual upbringing. While each religious sect provided its own interpretation of God, I felt the same love from God, regardless of the religion. When I felt stronger, I traveled back to the doctor in Little Rock for another breast MRI. I had to pay out of pocket, estimating my cost would be $12,000. I was surprised to learn my cost would only be $5,000, to which the radiologist said, "You realize this is a miracle." He proceeded to share the good news that the MRI showed the tumor had shrunk from eight centimeters to five millimeters, now the size of a small pearl. That was when I knew I was going to survive. I believed that all of my healing techniques were working together for the best outcome.

As I continued to heal, and the time for my surgery approached, my family and I talked a lot about the details. At dinner one night, my husband and I talked about what size my breasts would be once the reconstruction was complete. My appointment in a few days was with my plastic surgeon, and I would be learning about the different sizes and could see the implant samples. My daughter was listening and blurted out, "I want to go shopping with you for your new breasts!" We had a good laugh, and I decided to take her with me.

In the weeks just before surgery, a compassionate volunteer from Reach to Recovery came out to visit me. She was in her late sixties or early seventies. I asked her for her opinion on breast reconstruction and she said, "Oh honey, I don't use these anymore, so I didn't replace them." I replied that I had a thirty-two-year-old husband, and reconstruction was in my plan. I had been interviewing plastic surgeons and knew I wanted implants. Through my interactions with other female cancer patients, I learned that over 30 percent of men leave their wives during chemotherapy, surgery, radiation, or reconstruction. The stress of all the stages of cancer is real for both the patient and the caregivers. The treatment process definitely tests our emotional, physical, and spiritual strength. My goal was to make the most of the moment before my breasts were removed during my double mastectomy. I asked my husband, "Do you want to take pictures of these?" as I pointed to my breasts. I was willing to do anything to memorialize this moment in time and include him in the process. He smiled and nodded. We had a little celebration the night before my surgery, and he took photos.

Early on in my cancer journey, I was uncertain if my insurance would pay for a double mastectomy since my right breast was "healthy." Armed with the images from the cutting-edge breast MRI, which showed calcifications in my right breast, I was successfully able to negotiate with my insurance company to pay for the whole procedure. It is my understanding that a bilateral mastectomy is an insurance choice if your other breast is healthy. It is a personal decision and up to each woman to determine her choice given her own circumstances. There are no right or wrong answers.

I went to the hospital on October 2nd for my surgery. It was a seven-hour surgery, and all the lymph nodes on my left side were removed in the process. In addition, the plastic surgeon put expanders in place to hold the muscle for my reconstruction. I remember waking up in my hospital room and seeing flowers everywhere, along with my husband, mother, sister, and husband's business partner. I was thrilled beyond words to have woken up, to be alive! I looked down and saw ice packs on both of my breasts. It brought the reality of my situation back into focus. My husband stayed with me as I slept most of the day. Around midnight, I woke up in discomfort and looked down, noticing that my right breast and chest area were purple. I didn't know what was wrong, just that something was definitely wrong. I woke up my husband and asked him to get the nurse. All of a sudden, several nurses rushed in and quickly started preparing me for surgery. I guessed that it would take a while for surgery and asked my husband to call my sister so he would not be alone waiting and not knowing what was happening.

As soon as I was in the operating room, the surgeon discovered that I was bleeding internally. She had to suction everything out of my breasts, take out my expanders, clean out the area, and then put everything back. I ended up with over one hundred stitches per breast. Because of the emergency midnight surgery, I had a bigger scar on my right side than my left. Three days later, I went home with four drains, two on each side. A zip-up-the-front sports bra was the best recommendation another patient had given me prior to surgery, and I had brought one to the hospital. The sports bra held everything in place, and I could loop the tubes and pin them to my bra, keeping them close to my body. On October 19th, I was determined to attend my father-in-law's wedding, just a week after being discharged. I still had my drains and decided to wear a hat. I had been given two free wigs, but I found them to be very itchy and hot, so I didn't wear them.

The doctor recommended I massage my scars daily. I decided that was something I could engage my husband in, and he willingly agreed, in a very gentle way. I was determined to involve him in every step, helping him feel connected and giving him jobs to do, which helped him focus on something other than fear. My physical therapist recommended that I do exercises daily to help with my recovery. One of the exercises was "itsy bitsy spider" up the wall, which was fun to do with my daughter.

About a week after surgery, I went to the doctor for my breast expansion. I learned they used a magnet to find the entry to the expander breast in my chest. When my husband came home, I pulled some magnets off the fridge and started demonstrating what they did. We both laughed out loud, a deep belly laugh. At the time of surgery, I weighed only ninety-two pounds. The nipple reconstruction required extra skin and fat which I did not have, so I went with Barbie Doll mounds. My breasts didn't feel good in a regular bra for at least six months after my surgery, so I wore tank tops with a shelf bra. I was required to wait for several weeks post-surgery to heal before restarting chemotherapy infusions. I started again after Thanksgiving. Thankfully, my symptoms were minimal compared to pre-surgery. Since I was now in a state of "no evidence of disease," I no longer talked to the cancer.

Almost one year after my mastectomy, I experienced lymph-edema. I was working in the yard and I noticed my left hand was swelling a lot and my left arm was going numb. I called my doctor. He said, "This couldn't be lymphedema; it is a year later." I struggled to find resources on how to treat it. Finally, I found a therapist for lymphatic massage and drainage at a local hospital.

She taught me how to wrap my hand and arm and what exercises to do. I ordered a glove and sleeve to help with swelling. It took three months for the swelling to go down with lymph drainage massage, healthy eating, and gentle exercises. Through this experience, I learned that I really needed to be careful with my left arm and hand for the rest of my life, paying attention to swelling as a result of having no lymph nodes on that side.

Around the same time, I was enjoying dinner with my husband's entire family from New Orleans. Naturally, they were uncomfortable with asking me questions and didn't want to talk about my cancer experience. Our conversation seemed a little tense and sterile. All of a sudden, our daughter blurted out, "My mom doesn't have any nipples," which came seemingly out of nowhere.

I smiled and replied, "Yes, that is true." I felt grateful that the ice had been broken by my daughter calling out the big elephant in the room. We were able to switch subjects and enjoy the rest of the meal.

I experienced a strong support system and felt extremely fortunate during my entire treatment experience. I went back for a PET scan two additional times and had a CT scan every four months for eighteen months. During one of my visits, I wanted to understand the process at a deeper level. I asked the technician what he was injecting into me for the scan and how it worked. He said he put sugar in with the radiology fluid. Using the dye, the cancer was drawn to the sugar and became visible, like a flashlight on the scan. I filed that helpful information away and knew I wanted to stop eating sugar. After two years, I moved to one CT scan a year and at five years, I only had one if I had a severe complaint like a bad headache for three or more days. At ten years post treatment, I had an MRI because I was experiencing severe back pain. I learned that I had two bulging discs, which was more easily dealt with than a metastatic breast cancer diagnosis.

I was lucky to meet some amazing women during my treatment. I was determined to try to help other women who were facing breast cancer and provide support. Two other women and I founded Code Pink, a not-for-profit in Tennessee targeted for under-forty-year-old women with a breast cancer diagnosis, although any age woman was welcome to join, as cancer has no boundaries. One of my cofounders had been diagnosed while pregnant at thirty years old and had endured chemotherapy and surgery at the same time as I did. Our other cofounder's mother had died of breast cancer, and she became a nurse with a purpose. We outreached through word of mouth with our doctors. I personally spoke to over two hundred women and met with many of them at cafes around town. Within the first five years, twelve women had died from metastatic breast cancer, and our group gatherings began to dwindle. In our outreach, we realized 50 percent of the women stated they did not have any support system and about 30 percent of them lost their husbands to divorce during their battle. Cancer is a deeply traumatic experience for both the individual diagnosed and their loved ones, a roller coaster ride with many highs and lows. Each individual processes emotions and information in a different way, which leads to different experiences.

I survived each day during treatment by putting on my good soldier face and fighting the cancer. Through my treatment, I learned that it was good to be strong and have my armor, but also good to be vulnerable and let others help. I let people bring food, even when I could not eat it. I knew my family would be able to eat the food, or we could serve it to visitors. I felt that if I was saying no to any kind of help, it was like saying no to a friend. Friends would call and ask what they could bring. One time I replied, "I haven't had ice cream in a long time. If you bring ice cream, we can enjoy it together." That was a loving memory during one of my challenging days.

A friend of mine from college founded Planet Cancer at age thirty-one. She was diagnosed at twenty-six years old and wanted to create a digital support platform. Planet Cancer was the first website where young people talked about their lives and cancer, including the topics of sex, dating, and the trial drugs offered. Questions were addressed such as, "Do you tell someone on your first date that you have breast cancer?" I found her site amazing and helpful with camaraderie, and full of information about most any subject dealing with cancer, treatment, recovery, or terminal illness. She published a book in 2010 incorporating these experiences, called *Planet Cancer: The Frequently Bizarre yet Always Informative Experiences and Thoughts from Your Fellow Natives.*

As I reflect on my experience, it felt like all my friends wanted to be around me in the beginning while I was still learning details and processing all of my different emotions, which proved to be a difficult time to share because I felt stressed all the time. When I entered my recovery phase after my second chemotherapy treatment, I heard someone say, "Oh you look great. You look totally recovered!" In conversation with other survivors, I learned we were feeling similar thoughts, such as, *Oh really? I can't raise my arms more than halfway up. That doesn't feel like total recovery to me.* Putting myself in the other person's shoes, I realized that it was really no fault of theirs, as they had not experienced what I have been through and could not know. Recovery has no time frame, and from the outside, I looked normal. Each of us will experience something a little different and the timeframe could span years. It is truly a personal journey.

I look at recovery as the birth of the "new me." My family and I have been through a lot that changed us in many ways. My family, caregivers, close friends, and I each have our own interpretation and own story to tell about my cancer journey and the cancer-fighting team. The stories have similarities but can be very different in details. The "new me" has a positive twist to most scenarios, enjoying the little things with extra happiness, trying to fit as many activities as possible into any occasion. God presented me with many lessons during my journey. One of my cancer lessons was to "Never mind the annoying things and treasure the little things." In other words, ignore the little things that irk you, like getting stuck behind the garbage truck when you are in a hurry to get to your destination, but treasure the fleeting moments with your family, like picking out the perfect pumpkin at a pumpkin patch. If you surrender yourself in God's hands, he will liberate you spiritually from the weight of the cancer. I was liberated. It may not always seem like a positive outcome, but it is not always in our hands; we did our best to live a good life, fight cancer, and pay it forward.

During this journey, my first goal was to survive. I hoped and prayed, but never actually thought I would see our daughter graduate from kindergarten, so I wrote her letters. My second goal was to make it to five years, then ten years and now at seventeen years, I am inspired by those who are thirty years out. I see life from a different perspective. I am focused on the moment in front of me.

Advice for Others

How I supported myself
- I drank eight bottles of water a day from bottles marked "one" through "eight," to make sure I didn't miss one.
- I spoke to the cancer and told it to leave my body.
- I attended all the cancer groups, some several times, others only once.
- I engaged with other patients so we could support each other.
- I accepted help from all who wanted to help.
- I answered questions about treatment and cancer as they came up rather than locking away all the details of the journey, no matter how difficult.
- I tried to rest and sleep as much as possible.
- I tried to cut out as much processed sugar as possible from my diet.

How others supported me
- Friends and family brought food and even used the list that I had made for my husband as a guide of needs.

- Friends and family came to help with household chores—again, my list came in handy as they knew what needed to be done.
- Friends and family kept my daughter for overnights so I could attend certain appointments, such as PET or CT scans or surgery.
- I had a group of friends who came over for Game Night, since I was too weak to leave my home; I also stayed close to home for fear of catching an illness, which could potentially have been fatal with my compromised immune system.

Helpful tips

- Do not compare yourself to others: each journey is different, and someone else's story is a reference only.
- When someone is diagnosed with cancer, it is a normal part of the process to ask, "Why me?"
- Cancer is a roller coaster ride: it is normal to cry and then start laughing ninety seconds later.

TRICIA'S STORY

———— • ● • ————

It was May 2017, and I was breathing a sigh of relief, as I had just gotten through the end of school with my two daughters under the age of thirteen. I realized I was behind in scheduling my annual mammogram, so I called my doctor. I was able to schedule an appointment on May 22, using 3D mammography due to my previous experience with finding a lump. I was still adjusting to moving to a new city two years before and busy with life with two girls. I didn't consider the possibility that something might be wrong with me, as we were still struggling with our new reality related to my daughter's Type 1 diabetes diagnosis earlier in the year. In 2013, my mammogram had shown a spot that had led to a biopsy. The results had come back benign as it was just the dense fibrous tissue in my breasts. When I went in for the 2017 mammogram, the technician said she saw a spot. I said, "I'm not sure if I mentioned it, but this has actually happened to me before. A couple of years ago, I had a spot and it turned out clear. I am sure it will be fine." I scheduled the diagnostic mammogram and left thinking the outcome would be the same as before. I shifted to focusing on my family and diving into our summer fun, moving this topic to the back burner of my mind. I tried to live my life in the present, taking in the joys of each day. Hypothetical thoughts of a cancer diagnosis at this time would only depress me. On June 5, I went in for the diagnostic mammogram.

My phone rang a few hours later and it was the imaging center, calling me back and asking me to come in for a biopsy. I wondered, *How can this be? I am so broken with other things going on. This is nowhere on my radar, that something might be wrong.* Inside, I felt detached, as if this was someone else's story. I agreed, and we scheduled it for June 19, due to my busy schedule with summer activities. I went to the appointment by myself and was called back pretty quickly for the biopsy. I lay down on the table and met the doctor, then remember watching the biopsy needle going in. Despite the scary huge needle that looked like a harpoon, I watched the process on the radiologist's screen. I've always liked biology, and it was fascinating to watch the needle going in, and the tissue being taken; I was amazed by the new technology. The doctor finished and asked me to wait outside in the smaller waiting room to make sure she had all she needed. I sat down outside, remembering the harpoon needle and thinking, *This procedure was really stressful. I should have had a shot of tequila or taken a Valium before to help me relax. The process was emotional just by the sheer nature of the procedure.* I started talking to another woman who seemed scared and was about to have a biopsy. She was a mess. Since I had been through it before, I tried to comfort her. I was feeling positive that, although I was anxious, my results would turn out to be negative like before. The technician came out and said, "We've got the spot and you can leave. I will call you with the results in a few days." I let her know that I was leaving on a cruise to Mexico. She remarked, "Oh, I don't recommend swimming in the ocean after a procedure like this." I smiled and left, shifting my focus to packing and the trip.

I was preparing to go on a cruise with some girlfriends and was really excited. I was remembering that we had booked an excursion to swim with the whale sharks and thought back to the technician's instructions of not swimming in the ocean. I thought,

If I have cancer, too bad. I am going to live my life, go on the cruise, and swim with the sharks. Getting away and spending time with close friends gave me light and fed my soul, something I needed after the tough season we had just endured.

On June 21, 2017, the birthday of both my grandfathers, I drove to the airport to go on the cruise. My mom was in town to help with my kids, and she and my two daughters were in the car. My phone started ringing and I noticed it was the doctor. I answered, and she said, "There is no easy way to say this. The cells from your biopsy came back cancer. We think it is stage I. From here, you need to find an oncologist to develop a plan. You will have some decisions to make. Do you have a pen?"

I replied, "I am driving right now."

She said, "Oh my, I'm so sorry. I should have asked before saying anything. I would not have given you this news if I'd known you were driving a car." I told her I was leaving for a trip and would make decisions when I returned, and then we hung up. I knew I needed to keep my composure for the sake of my girls, as the shock of the results permeated my mind and my eyes filled with tears. Even with this news, I was committed to keeping my plans. It was a very special trip, planned by my maid of honor, and it was her treat. Both of her parents had died recently, her mom from breast cancer, and she was bringing her old roommates together to help bring joy back into her life. My mom knew that it was the doctor on the phone. She looked at me and mouthed the words, *You have cancer?* I nodded. My mom picked up her phone all of a sudden like she was on a mission and started texting my grandmother's best friend, who just went through something similar. She had chosen to have a lumpectomy and radiation, and never mentioned the diagnosis or treatment to any of her friends until after she was cancer free.

My mom looked at me and said, "Are you okay to go on this trip?"

I was determined and replied, as the tears now streamed down my cheeks, "Yes, I'm good to go. I'll be with my best friends. It's just three nights, and nothing is going to change in three nights. All of us have been so looking forward to this trip. These women will support me. I'm going."

My older daughter asked from the backseat, "Are you crying, Mom? What's going on?"

Given my daughter's recent Type 1 diabetes diagnosis, I wanted to be transparent and assure my daughters I would be okay. "Yes, I am. The doctor found a little spot of cancer in one of my breasts. They are going to do a small surgery to remove it, and I may need some treatment called radiation. I'm going to be fine. Mimi's best friend just went through it. She got through it, and so will I." My mom was very stoic sitting next to me; she was definitely not going to cry. I looked at her and said, "Right, Grammy?" and she nodded. My mind shifted to wondering, *Why is this happening now as we are still mourning the loss of my daughter's perfect health?* We had just lived through six months of change, including helping my daughter adjust, adding new steps to our daily routine, and fighting with the insurance to pay for all she needed. We were helping her test her blood sugar before every meal now, estimating her carbohydrates so we knew how much insulin to give her, and giving her insulin shots multiple times a day. I took a deep breath and shifted to acceptance mode, realizing that some things were going to happen the way they were going to happen, and they were out of my control. I thought of the saying, *What doesn't kill you makes you stronger*, but I was already feeling stronger without more on my plate to struggle with.

I hugged and kissed my mom and my girls, reassuring them that Mom would be fine and to have fun while I was gone. As I walked to get in the security line, I pulled out my phone to call my husband, who was at work. I said, "Hi, sweetie, how's your day?"

He replied, "Did the doctor call with your results?"

I said, "Yes. It isn't great, there is a tiny bit of cancer, although it is very early stage and treatable."

I could feel the fear in his voice when he said, "You have cancer?"

I replied, "I do, but my grandmother's friend just went through it. All I need is a lumpectomy and a few weeks of radiation. It is not a big deal." I was trying to minimize the diagnosis and downplay the impact.

His mind went straight to "living or dying," as his best friend's wife had died the year before of cancer, leaving him and a one-year-old child behind. He was still grieving deeply, and it was front and center for my husband and me every day. He said, "Where are you?"

I replied, "I'm at the airport."

He asked, "Are you really still going on this trip?" I told him yes, that nothing was going to change in three days, especially over a weekend.

I hung up and called my father-in-law, whose second wife had survived breast cancer. I said, "I need you. I am at the airport in line for security. I just found out I have breast cancer. I need you to tell your son it's going to be okay. I'm going on a trip and will find out more details when I get back." He agreed to help, and we hung up.

I made it through security and met up with one of the twelve women going on the trip at the gate. We hugged each other, and then I showed her the sombreros I had brought. We took some selfies, saying "Mexico or bust," as my phone lit up with a picture of my husband. He tried to convince me to not go and said he was at the airport. I explained, "Sweetie, I've already gone through security. I just got the results. When I get back, I'll have a bunch of tests, scans, and appointments to learn how big it is and what will happen next. I'll do a bunch of research and then we'll make decisions on what to do."

He said, "I just had to leave my office; this is a ton to process. Have you told our girls?"

I replied, "Yes, they were with me when I got the call, so they know. I need you be strong for them. They are going to have some questions for you about cancer. I don't want them worrying about me. I love you; it will be fine."

As I hung up, my friend who had just taken selfies with me said, "What's going on?"

I said, "You are not going to believe this. As I was driving here, I found out I have breast cancer. That's all I know right now." She wrapped her arms around me, which felt comforting and enabled me to focus on our trip instead of my diagnosis. I took a deep breath, and we boarded the plane to Houston.

I was shocked to learn how quickly word can spread now with the technology and devices we have grown to depend on. As I was on the flight, my husband was talking with one of my daughters, reassuring her that I would recover from my cancer. He didn't know that she was on the phone with a friend at the same time via FaceTime. Her friend overheard the conversation, told her mom, and within minutes, word that I had cancer spread like wildfire through my community, and everyone knew. When I landed in Houston, I had a message from my husband about the FaceTime story and lots of texts from friends. I immediately called the captain of my tennis team, who was my closest friend where I lived, hoping she had not heard the news before she heard it from me. Tennis was something I really enjoyed, and we had a close-knit team. She had already heard of my diagnosis, and I explained my situation, assuring her I would be fine.

As we walked off the plane, we met up with another friend who had landed before us. I caught her up on the story that was unfolding minute by minute. She reached out for my hand and said, "Oh, Tricia, you can beat this. It's no big deal anymore with the treatments and advancements the doctors have." I really needed to hear that and so appreciated her words of encouragement. My racing heart started to slow down. We met up with the rest of the group and drove down to Galveston the night before boarding the cruise ship. Each one of us had been roommates with my best friend, who had organized the trip. The drive went by fast as we all were telling stories and watching *Saturday Night Live* skits, laughing out loud. I felt my soul calming with each mile and each new story.

We arrived and checked into our hotel. One woman started making drinks as the rest of us put on sombreros, took selfies, hugged, and swapped travel stories. Someone had gotten stuck in traffic and almost missed her flight. Another woman said, "Oh that's terrible!"

I chimed in and blurted out, "Well, at least your doctor didn't call you on the way to the airport and tell you that you had cancer." There was a hush across the room, and you could have heard a pin drop.

My maid of honor looked at me and said, "Is that true?" I nodded as tears streamed down my face and reassured them I was going to get through it. I expressed how deeply I didn't want to bring negative news on our girls' trip, although it was where I was in the moment and not able to hide my feelings. I had just learned hours earlier of my stage I, HER2 positive cancer and it was taking up a lot of space in my head. The mood in the room shifted as the reality of the words I shared permeated our minds. Each of them hugged me, and I felt supported and loved. I convinced them to focus on the present and our amazing trip ahead of us. The next morning, we boarded the cruise ship and set out for our adventure. I was able to put my cancer aside and focus on where I was, building memories with close friends.

When I returned on June 24th, I started researching doctors and options for treatment, including referrals from my husband's best friend from his wife's experience. I interviewed ten survivors to learn their diagnoses and what they had chosen and found that each one selected a different type of treatment. Most of them recommended I have a double mastectomy, even though the tumor was only on one side. Hearing their stories was really helpful, and the knowledge felt like power over something I couldn't control. As I sat and thought about having surgery, I wasn't afraid. I had survived a head-on collision and had delivered my second child via caesarian section. I reminded myself that each of us is dealt a different hand, and I was going to embrace my situation, as I knew I was not the first to face this situation, and I knew I wasn't alone. Years earlier, I had served on an early childhood board in my community and was chair of the marketplace at our annual event. I was walking the floor of the event one day and a pillow caught my eye. I walked closer and saw the following scripture embroidered on the front: "For I know the plans I have for you, says the Lord, Jeremiah 20:11." I bought the pillow at the time as this verse really spoke to me. Here I was now facing a cancer diagnosis. I used the pillow through my treatment process as a helpful reminder to rely on God.

I ended up choosing an oncologist at an academic medical center. One thing I really appreciated about my experience was I could make any appointment at any office, and any doctor I saw had access to my records. The staff all seemed very happy in their jobs, which made the difficult experience more enjoyable. The oncologist ordered an MRI and took some blood for additional tests. When I went to meet the surgical oncologist on July 6, my husband came with me. He had several specific questions, and the doctor patiently answered all of them. Then she said, "So the tests results came back that there are two tumors in your right side, and you are actually stage II. You have a choice in terms of treatment—a lumpectomy with ten weeks of radiation or a mastectomy with no radiation. I am going to order some addi- tional tests and want you to come back tomorrow." Of all the survivors I had interviewed, the ones who had only had a single mastectomy had experienced a recurrence in the other breast. I remembered this and felt like having the lumpectomy or single mastectomy would keep me wondering every day if the cancer would come back. This felt to me like death by a thousand paper cuts. I told the oncologist I would think about it and get back to her. She also had me meet with a genetic counselor, as my aunt and grandmother both had breast cancer. I was told it would take a few weeks to get my results. On July 10, I called the doctor to let her know that I wanted to have a double mastectomy. She let me know that she would do a biopsy of my lymph nodes during the surgery, and the outcome would inform whether I would endure chemotherapy infusions.

One of the survivors I talked to who had been through the surgery recommended a bikini photo shoot before my surgery. She said she had done this and really appreciated having the pictures. It filled me with energy to think of capturing my body as it was before the surgery during a boudoir photo shoot, so I decided to do it. The photo shoot was a super helpful distraction from the many appointments and decisions related to my treatment. I chose to wear things that my best friends had given me and felt wrapped in love. It was fun and yet emotional, as I knew there was cancer growing in my body, and in a way, it felt like my body had failed me. The photographer had me hug my body in one of the pictures and I started crying, feeling my reality that part of my body would be removed and part of it had cancer. This picture remains one of my favorites in the album to this day.

Treatment Experience

Just before the surgery, I received a voice mail from the genetic counselor that I had tested negative for the BRCA gene, which surprised me given my family history. My double mastectomy surgery was scheduled for July 31, 2017 and my pre-operative appointment was July 27. I spent time alone leading up to the surgery, processing my reality as I was concerned. Knowing that this surgery would forever change a part of my body that was part of being a woman felt sad and heavy in my heart. I was also worried about my relationship with my husband, as I would have to wait for a while after the procedure to be intimate with him.

I was overwhelmed by the outpouring of love and support I experienced from my community, even strangers. A week before the surgery, I received a call from a woman whose son went to school with my daughter, someone I didn't know. She had heard about my cancer diagnosis. She had just been through a similar diagnosis and treatment. She walked me through what to expect and answered my questions. Hearing her advice and experience was helpful beyond words. On the night before my mastectomy, another woman pulled into my driveway in a pickup truck with a recliner in the back. She knocked on my door and said, "I heard you are having surgery tomorrow. I brought you something that you really need—a recliner." She was supportive and compassionate, telling me that I would beat it and that she would be there for me, although I didn't know her. Other friends brought over survivor socks that said "I am brave" on them, for me, my girls, and my husband. On the day of my mastectomy, my best friend in Southlake showed up to the hospital with lunch for my family, parents, and in-laws; then she stayed until I was out of surgery. The plastic surgeon put expanders in my breasts where the tissue had been to hold space for my implant surgery. My surgery went well, and I stayed in the hospital until August 2nd.

My husband had to pick up all the slack with our girls and household duties while I recovered post-surgery. This time period in our life put great stress on our whole family. While I recovered from my surgery, my oldest daughter was still trying to navigate all of the changes in her life from her diabetes diagnosis. I was still recovering when my girls went back to school, and I wasn't able to go or help out, which was something I enjoyed doing.

Several of my bridesmaids come in town to help me after the surgery, over two different weekends. One day while we were out shopping, my oncologist called while I was in the dressing room. She said, "I have your results from the tumors. You will not need to go through chemotherapy." I screamed inside, so excited, although I didn't want to cause a scene in the store. I waited until we were in the parking lot walking out to my car until I told them. We screamed and jumped up and down, hugging each other. I stopped at the store on the way home to get food and Champagne to celebrate. And I bought some napkins that said, "Best day ever."

I could feel the muscles in my neck start to relax as I sorted out what the words meant to me—no chemotherapy.

There are no words that would describe the deep feeling of love and support I felt from my close friends. One of them shared an article from wednesdaymorningwhispers.com about how elephants behave with other females in the herd: "Elephants take the formation of surrounding a female elephant when giving birth and when under attack. When our sisters are vulnerable, when they are giving birth to new life, new ideas, new ministries, new spaces, when they are under attack, when they need their people to surround them so they can create, deliver, heal, recover, we get in formation. We close ranks and literally have each other's backs." These friends sent me elephant pajamas and many other elephant gifts to remind me that they had my back. I was speechless and touched by their selfless acts of love.

Between my mastectomy and my transfer surgery on November 14, I would go back to the doctor every week or two so he could inject saline into the expanders, using a magnet to find the opening each time, similar to adding air to a balloon. He used a giant needle to inject the saline, which looked scary although I couldn't feel anything. I took a couple of friends with me to one appointment, and they were horrified at the sight of the needle. After my transfer surgery on the 14th, when the expanders were taken out and the implants put it, I felt tremendous physical relief, like, *Wow, I feel better.* All my breast tissue had been removed during the mastectomy, so my plastic surgeon wanted to do a third surgery to add fat tissue for appearances, which was February 1, 2018. Without the added tissue, my breasts looked like they had ripples similar to what a plastic bag looks like if you fill it with water. My final surgery was to take some fat from my stomach area, called my muffin top, to make it look like fat tissue versus an implant, a procedure called fat grafting. I ate pizza and drank beer for weeks before this surgery to build up enough fat. I woke up from the four-hour surgery in a compression outfit, still in pain. I had to wear it for three months. I could have opted for a fourth surgery to have nipples added and decided against that. I was done. My oncologist prescribed Tamoxifen and recommended I take it for five years.

My close friends in Southlake planned a pink party for my first birthday after the surgery, which was February 16. While this was not a "big" birthday as I turned forty-seven, it was significant as I didn't know that I would survive to see age forty-seven. My friend Liz had died of breast cancer despite having access to every possible treatment and doctor. If that had happened to her, I thought, it could happen to me. My friends who hosted the party also gave me a bracelet with a pink sapphire on it to commemorate the celebration. I stood up and thanked everyone, then gave a little speech about how it felt and what it meant to me to make it to age forty-seven, and thanked them for all of their love, prayers, and support.

Going through the cancer experience changed everything in my life and in my marriage. After the surgery, I felt less than. As my husband was younger than me, I was concerned how he would accept my butchered body. I had learned of a husband who had left his wife when she was diagnosed. I decided to face that conversation directly with my husband and told him he could leave me. He said no, he was committed to our marriage and was going to be around through the ups and downs. The cancer experience was felt deeply by my daughters as well. They had to adjust to Mom not being able to take them here or there or help with things when I was recovering. Something my older daughter, who was diagnosed with diabetes, said has still stuck with me to this day, "You get to have a surgery and your disease will go away, but mine is with me for life." As a mom, I was heartbroken hearing these words, wishing I could take away her diabetes, yet knowing I couldn't. One of the toughest side effects of taking Tamoxifen was my recall memory. My kids would get angry because I would forget things, which was hard to bear. In the big picture, I am grateful to have survived and have learned to live with my new body and the side effects from the medication.

Advice for Others

How I supported myself
- I prayed daily and thanked God for welcoming a new day.
- I listened to my body and rested when I needed to.
- I trusted God's plan every step of the way, whatever that was.
- I learned to accept gifts of service and say yes when people offered to help.
- I kept a gratitude journal where I listed what I was grateful for each day.

How others supported me
- I experienced bottomless support, acts of love, and gifts from bridesmaids, including doing laundry, cooking, and going grocery shopping.
- My tennis team wore baby pink uniforms and pink ribbons on their hats the whole season in my honor and would come over daily to check on me.
- I felt supported through countless phone calls, texts, and receiving cards in the mail from friends and family.
- I had so many people saying they were praying for me; I knew it made a huge difference.
- My community showed up in countless ways to support me.
- My survivor sisters shared their experience and helped educate me on the process.

Helpful tips
- While it may not be your intention, think about the conversations you have around people who have been diagnosed with cancer; talking about the worse-case scenario is not helpful, so be positive.
- Know that you never know what someone is going through; be compassionate and gracious.

- Know that the cancer journey is grueling and not a walk in the park; send a card or leave a voicemail rather than withdrawing from fear.
- No matter how well a cancer patient follows the treatment plan, there is still the unknown that is out of their control; life is a gift.

Helpful tips for cancer patients
- Take photos before surgery if your surgery will change how your body looks.
- Keep a journal, as the trauma of the experience impacts a cancer patient's ability to remember.
- Embrace the journey, take it one day at a time.

DEBI'S STORY

———— • ● • ————

In early December of 2015, I was working at a medical detox facility as the Activities Coordinator. It was a normal day as I headed out to Serenity Coffee Shop, which is owned by my friends and where I enjoyed going to lunch every day. I was sitting at a table waiting for my coffee. As my friend was walking over with my coffee, my left arm began to flop in front of me, and I felt dizzy. I looked up at him and said, "I think something might be wrong."

He stood next to me and asked, "Should I call nine-one-one?"

I said, "No thank you," because I thought it would stop. I called my best friend to come over. When she arrived, she knew something was wrong and said, "Which emergency room do you want to go to?" I could tell by her tone that it was definite we were going to the ER, and that part was nonnegotiable. I requested the one near my sister and brother-in-law's house, which was an hour away. The episode lasted about fifteen or twenty minutes.

As my best friend was driving me to the ER, I called my sister to tell her something strange had happened, like a seizure, and that I was heading to the ER near her. When I think back, I don't remember the drive or the phone call. Upon arrival, the nurse came out to get me right away and rushed me back. They thought I was having a stroke. I had one more episode when I was back in the room getting evaluated. The doctor ordered an MRI, and I was wheeled to the imaging room. The transitions were happening so fast it was hard to keep up. The technician asked, "Are you claustrophobic?"

I chuckled and said, "No, I've never been claustrophobic in my life."

She smiled, handed me a button, and said, "Well, if you change your mind, just push the button." Next thing I knew, the table I was lying on was carrying me into a narrow tube. Before the technician even started the machine, I pushed the button. The technician rolled me back out. I had begun to feel anxious, something I had never felt before.

We smiled at each other, and I said, "I think I do need a moment."

She said, "Don't worry, most people do." I lay there and prayed for several minutes, and then said I was ready to go back in, closing my eyes this time. As the loud noises banged around my head, I quoted scripture and prayed continuously. God brought me peace in the midst of the MRI. When the MRI was over, I was wheeled to a patient floor and admitted to the hospital. The doctor tried two different medications for seizures, but both made me dizzy and nauseated. He switched to a third medicine which I was able to tolerate. The nurse took blood and did an EEG and EKG. I went to sleep thinking I had experienced a seizure.

The next morning, I remember being woken up early by a doctor. It was December 8th. He introduced himself and then said, "Well I've got good news. You didn't have a stroke. The bad news is you have a brain tumor." He went on to explain what would happen next. He had contacted the neurosurgeon on call, and he was on his way to the hospital to read my MRI.

After the neurosurgeon read my MRI, he came by my room to explain what he had seen. He said, "Your tumor is on the outside of your brain, which is good. I can operate to remove it, and you won't need any additional treatment." The doctor made it sound like no big deal, so I took it that way. He said the hospital would make a follow-up appointment for me after I was discharged. Later when I learned more, I was grateful that this first neurosurgeon had conveyed the process like it was no big deal. It felt like protection from God and gave me time to process this information as I was still speeding through many transitions.

As I sat quietly, I heard God speak. He asked me, "Are you going to trust me?"

I answered, "Of course, I am going to trust you," like I felt I always did.

Then God spoke again and said, "No, I mean will you *really* trust me?"

I answered, "Yes, God, I will trust you."

I spent two nights in the hospital and was discharged the third morning. My best friend drove me, my sister, and brother-in-law to the surgeon's office for my appointment and called the office on the way to ask if we needed to bring anything. The person who answered the phone said no. When we walked into the doctor's office, the person behind the desk looked irritable and was short with us. She asked if I had the MRI disk and sharply said there would be no appointment if there was no disk. My bestie and sister felt frustrated, but I felt total peace and knew that was God intervening to guide me away from that doctor.

My best friend called my primary care physician and asked for a referral so I could get a second opinion. My doctor said he would try to reach a neurosurgeon he knew and call me back. He called back in a few minutes and said, "He is going to meet you in the ER in thirty minutes." We drove over to a new hospital and entered the second ER to meet the neurosurgeon my doctor had recommended. He read the MRI and said, "I agree your tumor is on the outside of the brain and probably operable, although I see a black spot that gives me pause. I would feel more comfortable referring you to an academic medical center, as they will be better equipped to handle your case. It's about three hours from here."

He continued to explain why this was important. Then he called for me and made the appointment, for the following week on December 17th.

I was taking the seizure medicine, which made me feel tired and dizzy. I wasn't able to drive and was not feeling well, so I had to request more time off from work. I spent a lot of time reading the word of God and praying. I felt the peace of God every moment and was not experiencing any fear. My sister and best friend were concerned for me and stayed by my side, providing great support during this time. My sister, best friend, and I made the three-hour drive the morning of December 17th for my appointment. The doctor introduced himself and explained what he was seeing on the MRI. He said the tumor was actually inside the brain and not operable. This took a moment to process, as two previous neurosurgeons had stated it was on the outside of the brain and was operable. He discussed the first step of treatment, an ablation procedure and a biopsy. Typically, he would have scheduled the procedure in two or three days, but since we lived so far away, he directed us to go to the ER so he could have me admitted that day. When I think back to the differences in opinions that three neurosurgeons had, I wondered how three doctors could look at the same MRI and all see something different. Later, when he came by my room in the hospital, I asked him. He explained that the other neurosurgeons focused on many areas of the body, but "I am the only one who specializes in the brain." I am confident this surgeon saved my life. As I heard the reality from the third neurosurgeon that the tumor was inside my brain, was not operable, and what would be required, I had complete peace from God and understood why God asked me if I was going to trust Him.

Treatment Experience

Within a day, my surgeon performed what's called an ablation procedure: he made a small hole in my skull and placed a thin laser probe in my brain. The computer screen showed him exactly what area was being heated and how much, making the treatment very precise. After the procedure, he explained my diagnosis, stage IV brain cancer, glioblastoma. He also explained that the prognosis was not good. I never cried or felt fear; instead, I began to get excited about going to heaven. I stayed in the hospital for four days and was able to go home on Christmas Eve. I never gave much thought to what things would be like after surgery, but from the moment I woke up, things had changed. I was no longer able to walk, and I needed twenty-four-hour care, as I couldn't do much of anything by myself. I don't remember much about the surgery, but I remember my three boys being there and the fun we were having together before the surgery, taking pictures. To have all three of my boys with me was worth a brain tumor.

I went to an oncologist after my ablation procedure to learn about my treatment plan. He recommended twenty-three months of chemotherapy and six weeks of radiation. Radiation and chemotherapy were only supposed to give me more time. Every time I had an MRI, the tumor was smaller than before. My youngest son ended up taking a semester off from college to take care of me. He came home for Christmas, and I made him go back to school for the spring semester. He was there two days when he called me and said, "I can't stay here, Mom. I want to be home with you." He came home and stayed with me for three months, taking care of my needs. I was most sad that I would not be able to see him get married. I ended up living longer than the doctor thought and was able to attend his wedding after all. My oldest son had my first grandson, who was born in April of 2016. I really wanted to be there for his birth in Texas. My doctor released me to travel, saying "Enjoy this trip because you won't likely get to go again."

At first, I took one chemotherapy pill a day every day for two months, then twice a day for five days a month. The drug regimen was extremely expensive, and my church paid for the first month. By the second month, the doctor had found a foundation to pay for the drug. When I first started my chemotherapy treatment, I was sick for the first day, feeling nauseated and listless. The doctor was able to change my anti-nausea medicine, and I felt good from that day forward. Radiation was every day during the week for six weeks, and I mostly felt tired. After nine months, the tumor no longer showed up on the MRI.

Once my brain cancer treatments were complete, I discovered a new issue, a lump on my breast. I called my primary care physician, and he ordered a mammogram. An hour after I had the mammogram, he called me and asked me to come into the office. I knew that was not a good sign, although I wasn't worried. When I arrived, he sat down and said, "I saw the lump, and by the shape of it, I think it's malignant. I would recommend you see an oncologist and get it checked out." Interestingly enough, a primary cancerous brain tumor cannot spread elsewhere in the body, so this was unrelated to the brain cancer. My neurosurgeon referred me to an oncologist for my breast tumor. He did more diagnostic tests, including more specialized mammograms, and determined I needed a biopsy. When the pathology came back from the biopsy, the specialist said it was stage I, and I would probably just need a lumpectomy.

After my lumpectomy, the pathology came back as stage II and then I had to go through both chemotherapy and radiation again. During each step of this process, I was calm, never getting discouraged and always saying, "I trust God and my path. I know it is for my good and His glory." Thankfully, I did not get sick from the chemotherapy this time, although I was very tired. The worst part was a shot I received the day after each chemotherapy treatment called Neulasta. The shot was supposed to boost my white blood cells, but it caused bone pain in the process. For me, this was excruciating pain, landing me in the ER some days. To my surprise, I learned that taking Claritin was a way to avoid the bone pain—yes, the antihistamine. My best friend and I laughed as we pondered who figured that out. It was funny, well, once the pain stopped anyway. I quickly discovered the generic didn't work and I had to take the brand name Claritin. I take a pill now to suppress my estrogen levels and have to continue it for the next five years.

When I saw my neurosurgeon after my treatment was complete, he said, "I love your attitude, it's the reason you're still here."

I said, "No, it's my God." My MRI showed no evidence of disease. God has taught me the difference between trust and appreciation through this experience. I learned that when I trusted God in the good times, it felt more like appreciation. And when I trusted God in the hard times, it felt to me like faith. I teach a Sunday school class at church, which I started before my diagnosis, called "When Life is Hard." God is good all the time, even when it doesn't feel good or look good. I have found countless blessings and opportunities through this experience, including bringing all three of my boys home, and I am in awe with the joy I feel. I have learned so much and grown through this season of despair and pain. While I grew up a fairly judgmental person, this experience has made me more accepting of others. I want to be like Jesus—if it takes cancer to be my best self, bring it on.

I wasn't able to drive for the first year after my ablation. A group of friends got together with a nonprofit organization called Ride for the Fight and bought me a golf cart so I could get around the neighborhood. It was such a blessing to be able to have some freedom from being indoors and the ability to get around in my community. Another group of friends from my neighborhood held a fundraiser for me, which enabled me to pay my ongoing medical bills, and my church provided support through meals. It was amazing to watch the body of Christ come together. I was humbled and felt so very blessed. A Bible study group took up a collection to pay for my food when I traveled to the doctor. Ride for the Fight paid for my lodging and gas when I had to travel to treatment.

I was stable for three and a half years until August 30, 2019. My legs started to grow weak, and after a week, I could barely walk. At this point, my best friend took me to the ER. Going to the emergency room this time was different because I knew something wasn't right. I was walking differently, doing things differently, and not very physically stable. Yet, at the same time I'd had so many clear MRIs that I was almost surprised at the report. I don't know why I was surprised it wasn't clear, but I was. A CT scan revealed inflammation in my brain, so I was admitted overnight. I had an MRI in the evening and was told the next morning that there was a new lesion in my brain. I knew the next step was to call my neurosurgeon—I trusted him with my life. He had me come down that morning and prepare for another ablation, which I had on September 7. This time the ablation affected my speech and my whole right side. As such, I was transferred to an acute rehabilitation hospital, where I stayed until I was discharged on September 26. Rehabilitation was a new experience for me, and I pushed through the challenging exercises each day, wanting to get better.

This new season in my life has been hard, but God has been at work even here, letting me speak about Him. Now that I am home, I am unsure what is going to be permanent and what is going to get better in my walking and my talking, but God will get me through it. The journey is not over until I'm in heaven, and it's going to be a great journey no matter what happens. The great news is I learned in late September 2019 that the mass in my brain is not a tumor and not cancer! The lesion is reactive glioma, which is caused from radiation. Post-surgery treatment included steroids to reduce the inflammation in my brain, antiseizure medications, physical therapy, and an MRI in one month. Hopefully, prayerfully, as the inflammation in my brain subsides, my ability to walk will improve.

Even when the MRI came back with a new lesion, I had peace. I've always had peace. I've never had an ounce of fear through this whole thing, and I didn't when I went to the hospital or when he did the ablation. I just wasn't scared. I know in my head I probably should have been, but I was not. God gave me the grace that I needed to endure all that I have, and that's the only way I can explain. People I share this story with say how strong I am, and if only he or she could be that strong given the same experience. But, it's not me, it is *God*! If they were going through it, they would have the choice to either accept God's grace in the journey He wants or not . . . which, by the way, has been the best journey of my life. I've told three people just today in the last three and a half years I've had a brain tumor, gotten divorced, and had breast cancer. It has been the best three and a half years of my life. They look at me and don't even know what to say except, *Wow, I wasn't expecting you to say that*. But, as Christians, God chooses our journeys, and if we're not living in sin and we're listening to Him, our journeys can be great. We can know that it is all for our good and His glory! I plan to walk this journey however long it lasts. If I die tomorrow or I die in ten years, my trust level is not going to change. I am going to trust God and it's a win-win.

These days, my conversations with God are more like *Come teach me and grow me*, and *Thank you for this journey*, and *Whatever you have in store for the future, I'm here, I'm ready to go*. I'm going to be obedient. I'll do it every day until I get to heaven, which is a win-win. There's no losing for me.

Advice for Others

How I supported myself
- I prayed daily and read scripture, talked to God.
- I listened to praise music and focused intently on the lyrics to help me heal.
- I filed for disability and was amazed at how little I was able to live on, and how happy I was.
- I chose joy every day.

How others supported me

- My sister, sons, and my best friend were with me through every step, supporting me with unconditional love.
- The church and the community I live in took up collections for food and paid for our hotels and gas for our trips to the academic medical center three hours away.
- I have received checks in the mail from people I had not talked to in a while for the exact amount I needed at the time to pay bills.

Helpful tips

- Trust that God is good and get past "why me, why now"; it may look bad, but it is not bad.
- Whatever happens, God has handpicked you for this journey you are on.
- Know that if God has allowed it, it is for your good and His glory.

ALAN'S STORY

———•●•———

It was early February of 2010, and my wife Amy had been com-
plaining about pain in her legs, in the area where her lymph
nodes were. She had recently bought some new shoes and decided
it must be the shoes, as it couldn't be something wrong—she was
never sick. A few weeks went by and the pain continued. The focus
for us shifted, though, as Amy's dad died suddenly of a metastatic melanoma tumor in his brain on February 13. We traveled
to Knoxville for the funeral and returned to Nashville, grieving
deeply for a beloved man. Amy felt lost without him and walked
around most days in a fog. She did her best to keep it together for
our three children, who were under the age of twelve.

A few weeks went by and the pain was still there. I encouraged her to go to the doctor. She saw her primary care physician,
who examined her and was concerned about the location of the
pain. He said pain in her lymph nodes was a signal of something
else. He ordered an MRI and had the nurse take some blood.
Despite Amy's family history with her dad dying of melanoma,
Amy had never had any issues. She had had a mole removed nine
months earlier that was benign. A few days later, her doctor called,
and she immediately called me at work and said, "Honey, I have
some news although I am still in shock. My doctor just called. I

have stage IIIC metastatic melanoma." She stopped for a minute and silence filled the air as we both sorted out these heavy words. She continued with more details, and I agreed to come home from work. The MRI showed the lymph nodes were affected, and he said some needed to be removed. She was forty years old. That conversation when she shared the news will be forever etched in my memory, as it was the beginning of our lives changing forever.

We sat our children down when they came home from school later that day to tell them. We had agreed to be straightforward with them. Amy did an amazing job—she was matter of fact and laid out what she had learned plain and simple. She calmly explained that she had cancer and described where it was and what the doctors would do to remove it. We let them know she'd be in the hospital for a while and then she would be recovering at home until she was better. We didn't talk about mortality rates or risks, although we both knew she only had a 20 percent chance of living another five years. We wanted to be honest with them but didn't want to scare them. Our youngest son was too young to really grasp what Amy was saying. The older two were stunned and quiet, and then moved on to how it would affect them. My oldest son said, "Who will take us to school and to soccer practice? Is Grandma coming to help?" They were brave but worried. We did our best to reassure them that we were doing all we could to get Amy the best treatment possible. In an effort to shift back to normal life, we took them to a Predator's hockey game that night.

It was a month after we had laid her dad to rest, and Amy was a mess. She made the drive to Knoxville to tell her mother in person about her diagnosis. As she drove that day, it was raining. She was really questioning God and why he had taken her dad just a few short weeks before and now she had been diagnosed with cancer. It was way more than one person should have to experience in a lifetime. She called me from the car and said, "Hey, Alan, so you know how we have been questioning God lately? Well I was just questioning God again. And all of a sudden, I drove through a wide patch of colors all around me in the middle of the highway, near the Cumberland Plateau. I thought I was imagining things, and then I drove through another one. I figured out they were the ends of rainbows from the storm. I have never seen anything like it before. There were at least four of them, and suddenly everything seemed clear to me—though there was a storm, there could still be beauty and rainbows. I pulled over, and a waterfall of tears poured from my eyes. I am still sitting here, in awe of God's timing and miracles." As we were hanging up, she reassured me that she had not lost her mind, that she thought it was an answer from God and wanted me to believe it as well.

Her doctor scheduled her surgery with a surgical oncologist for mid-April of 2010 to remove "quite a few" lymph nodes in her right groin, pelvis, and abdominal area. The doctor said it was clear that she needed surgery, although the treatment path afterward was less clear. The pathology of the lymph nodes would inform her treatment plan, which she would develop with an oncologist following surgery. Amy started capturing her cancer journey on CaringBridge, which helped her process and gave friends and family a vehicle to get updates in a streamlined way. Amy was a computer science major and had worked in the software industry. She started using CaringBridge because she was getting annoyed by constantly having to reply to emails and texts asking how she was doing. The problem with CaringBridge is that it wasn't search-able, at least not in 2010. Later on, as she started clinical trials and experimental drugs, she moved her writing to a blog on WordPress, nashvegasmom.wordpress.com, so other people trialing the same drugs could read of her experience and learn about side effects, in an effort to help them.

We knew there was a high probability of the cancer recurring and wanted to take the most aggressive, proactive steps we could to beat the odds. We started widely researching treatment options, as she was willing to go to great lengths to survive. We were not satisfied with what our local academic medical center was offering, so we started researching leading cancer centers in other states. We found a clinical trial for biochemotherapy at a leading cancer center in Houston that looked promising. Amy called and was able to gather all the details, including timelines and deadlines.

We had adopted a puppy a week before Amy's dad died, before Amy was diagnosed, as our other dog had died of lymphoma over the holidays. This new puppy was a handful as we attempted to housetrain her, and we would find her chewing on something not meant for dogs every time we turned around. In the midst of our chaotic life, our dog was diagnosed with mange a week before Amy's surgery. I told Amy that we should send her back to the shelter, as it was more than we could handle given our new life circumstances. She replied, "Oh, Alan, that sounds like a country song—my Grandpa died, my mom has cancer, and they sent my puppy back. All we're missing is a ramshackle pickup truck! I won't hear of it, we're keeping her." We both started laughing, deep belly laughs, as we thought of the start of our new country song. I reassured her we would keep the puppy.

As we arrived for her surgery and she was being prepped, she asked the surgeon, "So, how many lymph nodes are you going to remove today doctor?" He changed the subject and joked around, saying, "I have to pull everything out of there, dig out the lymph nodes, and put it all back." Having never been sick and having only been to the hospital to give birth, Amy didn't think this surgery would be that bad. She was sadly wrong and ended up with two large incisions, three drains, and a six-day hospital stay. She really struggled with digestive issues and thought she would never be able to eat again. When she was in her room, the surgeon came by to explain what he had found. "A few lymph nodes" turned out to be thirty-seven, fourteen of which were cancerous.

She left the hospital wearing a compression stocking on her right leg from hip to toe, with instructions to wear it every day to control the swelling. Amy was able to keep her spirits up most days, and whenever she felt her mind slipping to that deep dark abyss of what might happen next, she would employ one of her emergency tactics. These included saying a Hail Mary, as we are Catholic, or playing Prince's "Let's Go Crazy," though not at the same time. She was a brutally honest and independent woman, but she knew that cancer was bigger than she was. Her time spent in prayer increased as her journey progressed, mostly due to the rainbow sighting.

Scheduling new appointments with oncologists quickly is tough to accomplish; thankfully Amy had two friends who work in offices trying to help from the inside. Amy told them, "When they hear how smart, funny, and doggone special I am, they'll clear their calendars for me!" That was Amy, very witty and sarcastic at the same time. Amy's witty nature was one of her gifts that always made me smile and drew me closer, deepening my love for her. We were able to get an appointment in the middle of May with an oncologist, thanks to our friends' help.

As we waited for the appointment, Amy recovered from her surgery and stayed focused on being an involved parent, helping with homework, and driving our kids to school and activities. The day finally came for her appointment, and we were eager to talk about her treatment plan with her oncologist. He was empathetic, easy to understand, and really took his time. We really liked him and his transparency, so we knew what we were dealing with. He shared the news that based on the pathology of the lymph nodes, she only had a 20 percent chance of surviving five years. This was not new information for us, as the day she was diagnosed, we both Googled "stage III melanoma prognosis," and saw the same odds. While we both knew them from day one, we never discussed them.

Our lives were definitely turned upside down from this day forward, like a roller coaster ride with periods of calm and bursts of change. The oncologist recommended radiation and was supportive of the biochemotherapy treatment we had found. Amy had a strong will to live, if not for herself, for our three children. She was a dedicated mom, who had chosen to give up her job to be around shortly after our daughter was born. Later that day, Amy was able to schedule an appointment for May 27th at the leading cancer center in Houston for the biochemotherapy treatment. This was day fifty-two of the "start treatments within sixty days of surgery" deadline she had been given by her doctor. A few days later, we went to the radiation oncologist, who explained the process and recommended three weeks of radiation, with a plan to start in two weeks.

The following Monday, Amy had a PET scan and a CT scan. Her doctor called her the next day with the results, announcing that there was no sign of cancer. The spots that had shown on her left side lymph nodes were gone. When I came home from work, we hugged and screamed, celebrating this great news. Then she said, "I wish I had time to go to medical school or retake my high school biology class. It's hard to know what to do. I pray we come back from Houston a week from today with a clear path forward for treatment." She and I talked about how much had changed in our lives in a few short months since her dad's death. She tried to stay positive despite the hand she had been dealt. She said, "My life is no different than anyone's. There are no guarantees. None of us knows when the end will come. Shouldn't we all be living today like it's our last?" I decided that my positive attitude had perhaps influenced her outlook a little.

On Wednesday morning, she met with a lymphedema therapist to have her leg wrapped for the flights to and from Houston. Going into the appointment, she was expecting an Ace bandage, but she came out looking like she had a full leg cast, right down to her toes. We had to stop at Target to buy a sandal she could wear with this new addition to her wardrobe. Amy's mother came in town to take care of our kids, and we headed to the airport, getting through security quickly and boarding the plane. During the flight to Houston, Amy said, "I look at the life you and I have built around us in sixteen years of marriage—our friends, our faith, our family—and all of a sudden I see such power and strength. It has brought me such peace, even though I am facing this cancer and treatment."

After we landed in Houston, we drove to the cancer facility within the medical center and were shocked by the sheer size of the block after block of hospitals and specialty centers. It was staggering and not something we had seen before. As we waited outside, we looked at each other, and I said, "This reminds me of Disney World. There are shuttles in and out—every hotel you can name, with lost travelers wandering around to get their bearings. Only these tourists are limping and bald, with bandages and wheelchairs."

She smiled and said, "Yes, I thought the same thing. Welcome to Cancer World."

When we met with the doctor, he was compassionate and upbeat. We learned he was the deputy head of the department, which reassured us. He told us that he had patients with Amy's diagnosis coming in for their ten- and fifteen-year checkups. Finally, some hope from a doctor! Amy went through a series of rigorous tests, and then the doctor recommended a plan which involved going back to Nashville to complete radiation and lymphedema therapy for the swelling in her leg, and then returning in a month to Houston for treatment. She would be in Houston for a week to get infusions in the hospital, go home for two weeks, then start again three more times, for four total treatments.

On our plane ride home, we felt relieved that the pieces were falling into place and that she had a treatment plan. She was so ready to get going and start something, it didn't matter how small. She looked at me and said, "It scares me to imagine you juggling your job, summer vacation with three kids, and me hobbling back and forth to Houston. I do believe the Lord will help us through this, just as He has finally shown us the path He wants me to take with this illness. I feel Him every day through everyone around me." Amy was raised Methodist but didn't go to church regularly and didn't grow up in a very religious home, as her dad was a firm atheist. She chose to join the Catholic Church after we got engaged because she liked that it was such an important part of my family's life and identity. She was about as religious as anyone else you'd meet, but the cancer journey changed all of that. It gave her something to hold onto. Her faith became an anchor for her.

Treatment Experience

On Tuesday, June 1, she started the first of her seventeen radiation treatments, as well as lymphedema therapy for the swelling in her leg in Nashville. For radiation, she went every weekday for three weeks, plus two days the fourth week. Her main side effects from radiation were nausea, some burned skin, and fatigue. Her doctor gave her medication for the nausea, which helped. On her way down to the waiting room at the hospital for a radiation treatment during week two, she and I walked slowly next to a much older gentleman. He shuffled along with his gnarled left hand wrapped in an old cotton garden glove, discussing the nearly two-hour wait we'd had. He told us he'd already had five hours of chemotherapy that day. Then out of the blue, he said, "This wasn't in my plans. I'm supposed to be fishing." Amy told me later that it was as if her dad had reached right out and spoken to her, as if these words were from him. It rang so true for her, like a church bell. Cancer was not in her plan either, and yet here we were. When the radiation was finished, she had a week or so to recover, and then she had a cardiac stress test and a pulmonary function test to ensure she could withstand the treatment protocol in Houston. Fortunately, both tests came back normal.

We arranged for my mom to take care of our children and flew to Houston on July 5, after celebrating Independence Day with our family. On the 6th, she underwent general anesthesia to have the port-a-cath installed near her clavicle. The biochemotherapy infusions started on July 8th and were to be administered for a week in the hospital in Houston; then we would travel home for two weeks of recovery and repeat three times. The drug regimen was a nasty cocktail of Cisplatin, Dacarbazine, Interleukin 2, and Vinblastine. It was a controversial treatment, but we believed it was the best option for her. It was the most aggressive treatment available, but it felt right to us, as she had a very rare mutation of melanoma that was tough to treat.

Amy said she felt mostly like she had the flu with continuing nausea, chills, fever, and a lack of appetite. She slept most of the day. She kept a picture of our children next to her bed and stared at it when she was awake, as she deeply missed them. On day four, Amy and I were able to go outside and walk down to the butterfly garden. We were the only ones outside and would have stayed longer, except the Texas heat and humidity hit us hard. We got back to the room and Amy noticed her face in the mirror and said, "Hey, I kind of look like Violet from *Charlie and the Chocolate Factory!*" We both laughed, bringing some levity to a situation that felt overwhelming. Humor became a very helpful coping mechanism as we walked this scary and unknown path together. I stayed by her side the whole time, trying to keep her positive despite her side effects. While we were in the hospital, we met a couple from a small town in Arkansas, who had three boys. They were big University of Tennessee fans like us, and we really bonded. The mom was on the same treatment as Amy and the same schedule. As we were preparing to be discharged, the nurse gave Amy a Neulasta shot to help boost her immune system. She also told Amy that her side effects had been minimal compared to other patients. We felt that the minimal side effects were a result of the many prayers from our family and friends.

We flew home on July 14, delighted to see our children. Amy had a comforting place to sleep and recover before we turned around and did it again in two weeks. Amy's oncologist had recommended she consider buying a wig in case her hair fell out, which had about a 30 percent probability. She hadn't really thought much about hair, and compared to trying to survive, losing her hair seemed trivial, she had said. A week after we returned from Houston, Amy's hair started coming out faster than her normal rate. She said, "So, Alan, it suddenly doesn't feel like 'just hair' anymore. I really like my hair. I'm glad I have a lot of it, but I think I need a trip to the wig shop soon. My friend suggested getting two wigs, a blonde one for 'fun Mom is here' and a red one for 'don't mess with Mommy.' What do you think?"

That was Amy, always trying to turn something tough into humor so she could cope. I told her that sounded great, whatever she wanted was fine with me. She decided to get a scarf instead of a wig, as she liked it better. Although her hair was thinning, she had so much of it that it was not noticeable to others. She then announced confidently that she was going to be among the minority of survivors of stage IIIC melanoma at least ten years from now, as she had three children to embarrass. Her deepening of her faith, along with my positivity, guided her belief in her ability to survive, and I was delighted to hear it.

We flew back to Houston for round two, and Amy was feeling strong and ready, as it meant she was half-way through the infusions. When we had been there two weeks earlier, Amy had made a bold fashion statement by parading around the halls with her IV pole in her sock monkey pajamas. As we walked by the gift shop on our way to her room, we noticed they had changed the display case in the front window. It was now full of sock monkeys! Was that a coincidence? I didn't think so. We also saw the couple from Arkansas again. While our wives slept, her husband and I would go grab dinner together. Toward the end of her infusions, Amy was really weak and needed a blood transfusion. I was frustrated that I wasn't able to donate for her as it took twenty-four hours to process and they wanted to do it quickly. I made a mental note to donate when we first arrived the next time just in case. She experienced symptoms similar to the first time, although at an increased intensity. She survived the infusions, and we were able to return home as scheduled. When Amy was feeling better after several days, she looked at the calendar and realized her third treatment was scheduled for the first week of school. She called her doctor and pushed out the start of the third infusion for another week. She really loved being a mom and wanted the full back-to-school experience, complete with driving each child to school and taking first day pictures of them.

As we prepared ourselves mentally and emotionally for the third trip, she remembered something her doctor had said months ago. She said, "Melanoma is not the kind of cancer where you reach five or ten years and your odds go back down to the same as everyone else. It's the kind where you hear, 'Come back when you're stage IV, and there are lots of things we can try.'"

I wrapped my arms around her as these words permeated our minds, knocking down our optimism a little. I looked at her and said, "You are going to beat this. And I am going to be by your side every step of the way." Amy smiled and we hugged again. She was happy to have a semblance of normal life with back-to-school shopping and being able to drive. We then organized our life at home again in order for us to step out of it and head to Houston for another round.

She started with a full body PET scan and a CT scan before the infusions. Both came back clean, which we celebrated by dancing around her room. The third infusion was similar to the second and she did end up with more blood transfusions. All in all, Amy endured the poison seeping through her veins well with limited side effects. We were able to come home as planned, she recuperated as before, and we were able to attend ordinary events, such as soccer games and guitar lessons. All in time for round number four.

As we arrived for the last week in Houston, we ran into the Arkansas couple again. We talked about the situation we were each facing, both being dealt a hand of facing eternal rest at way too young an age, and both women fighting with everything they had to survive. We made a commitment to stay in touch after the treatments. Later when we were back in Amy's room, the nurse came in and declared that the last bag of drugs was empty, and she was done. Amy and I looked at each other, in part in shock that it was over and in part feeling huge relief that it was over. Over the previous six months, the surgery, radiation, biochemotherapy, and five hospital stays had drained us of the many joys of daily life that we had taken for granted before the diagnosis. We were staring at each other in disbelief of all we had endured.

A few minutes later, we heard the news come on from the television across the room and turned to look. The weatherman was showing a picture of the Houston skyline, announcing that an enormous rainbow was arching from somewhere outside of the city, off camera, with the end of the rainbow landing right on the medical center where we were. We looked at each other, stunned by the similarity to the one on her drive six months earlier. She looked at me and said, "Alan, I know where the other end of this rainbow is. It's on the Cumberland Plateau. And while you know I have never been an evangelical type or believed in the supernatural, this is not something we can explain away or ignore. It's a sign for us that God can do amazing things in the midst of our pain; all we have to do is ask." I wrapped my arms around her as tears poured down both of our cheeks.

When we returned to Houston in late October 2010, the doctor announced that there was no evidence of disease on her scans. She was to continue having scans every three months in Nashville. We started planning a family celebration to memorialize the occasion. Our nine months of nightmare were over, and we were on the other side. We were all delighted to be able to celebrate Christmas with Amy there, not something we were certain of just a few short months before. We dove into our busy lives with our three children and celebrated normal days of carpool and standing on the sidelines of track meets and soccer games. After the first of the year, we made some tough decisions. We decided to move our three children to a Catholic school. Amy really felt strongly that this school would be a place for them to thrive and be grounded in faith, whether she was around or not. We also decided to sell our beloved home and move to a neighborhood close to the new school. Preparing for these transitions and buying a new house kept us busy, in addition to living life with three young children.

In April of 2011, following her quarterly full body scans, the doctor called to say a spot had shown up in her right hip, in the ball and socket. It was very small, and the doctor decided to watch it, as he said it could be something other than cancer. We both talked about it and decided to hold the positive space and affirm that it was not cancer. When we went back in July, the spot was still there, and it had grown. She was now considered stage IV. We were both devastated and speechless, as we had been so hopeful that we had beaten this, and that life would be back to normal. After all she had gone through in Houston, it felt like a punch in the gut—a death sentence. Afterward came some really dark days for us, in which she did better than I at maintaining her faith after this terrible news. I was angry.

The orthopedic surgeon started planning for surgery to remove the spot in her hip, which was August 9. Amy was insistent on moving quickly to surgery and felt like it was important to get the cancer out of her body as quickly as feasible. It was major surgery, where he would remove all the muscles in her lower hip and buttocks area on her back side, drill a hole in the back of her pelvis, scoop out the tumor with a melon baller-like device, fill in the space with bone cement, and then reattach all of her muscles. The surgeon also put a plate and some screws in to strengthen her pelvis. As it turned out, the surgery was scheduled the day before the move to our new house. I knew we needed to have Amy distracted and away from the move, or she would have tried to help. She was in the hospital for three days, which gave us time to get moved in and her time to rest. Our new house was a ranch style, which we knew we needed after the surgery, and she came home with a walker.

Amy was delighted to experience another back-to-school week with our children, complete with photos—one of her favorite times as a mom. She gained strength every day and graduated from a walker to a single crutch. She went for another round of radiation on September 7 with a plan to go twice a day, six hours apart, every weekday for two to three weeks. This was risky as she had already had radiation on the same area and was getting close to her lifetime maximum. It was a risk she wanted to take to give her every chance of success. She experienced the same skin-burning and fatigue side effects, although this time the radiation didn't cover any of her organs, so she didn't experience nausea.

On the first Sunday of her radiation, we went to Mass at a local church near our new house. The priest asked for anyone who was ill or undergoing surgery to come forward and be anointed with holy oil and receive a special blessing. Here was a perfect opportunity for Amy, although she froze in the pew and didn't move. She was actually a very shy and private person, although her cancer experience was changing that. When I asked her why later, she said fear had taken over. We talked about how that experience was likely purposefully put in her path. The next morning during her rosary, she prayed for God to put her back in the place of trust again where she had been a few weeks earlier. When she finished, her phone started ringing. It was a priest from our children's Catholic school asking if he could come over and anoint her with holy oil and pray—a direct response to her prayer. He came over when all of us could be there and prayed for Amy to trust in God and for Him to give her patience and heal her. A few weeks later, on October 4, the scans once again showed no evidence of disease (NED).

We enjoyed a thrilling Thanksgiving and Christmas holiday season in the NED state, getting to enjoy the daily joys of life and feeling somewhat normal spending time with family, despite Amy's permanent limp. As we entered 2012, I could see Amy's anxiety increasing as she was due for her first quarterly scans. A couple of spots lit up on the PET scan, which once again deflated our bubble of joy and hope. It set Amy back to square one, feeling afraid of what might happen next. The oncologist ordered follow-up tests and blood work and, on January 17, ordered us to "Go out and celebrate. No evidence of disease and no tumors. We will see you again in three months."

Amy and I went to dinner to celebrate. We knew that the roller coaster that had become our life could shift again at any moment. She looked at me and said, "You know, Alan, I am relieved with the news. The reality is we all live with a death sentence that is unknown in its length. This cancer has really given this awareness to me. It has also freed me, and I feel like my choices are amplified. As we approach the second year of this journey, it is really clear to me that what I want most is to live and take care of our children."

And sure enough, the roller coaster ride took a turn for the worse just a week later. Her MRI showed a very small tumor in the right ventricle of her heart. We were relieved that the cardiologist caught it, as Amy's oncologist couldn't even see it, which is why she had been declared NED. We met with the oncologist the following week and determined that he would repeat the CT and MRI scan in two weeks to see if the tumor had grown. There were two new melanoma drugs that had just been approved, Yervoy and Zelboraf, and he had planned to use Zelboraf first to shrink the tumor. Despite the deep frustration of the ups and downs, Amy was determined to fight, fight, and never give up. The funny story is when they first told us about this new drug, it didn't have a commercial name yet. We offered up some suggestions like "mela-no-more" and were disappointed to hear they ignored our input and went with Zelboraf. That was classic Amy, always using humor.

On April 18 she started on Zelboraf, which was a pill she could take at home. It sounded like a promising drug that targeted one particular part of the cancer cell and stopped it from growing out of control, while leaving the healthy cells alone. On day two, she was experiencing nausea, fatigue, dizziness, and fever. We continued with our normal activities and even traveled to see our daughter play in a soccer tournament the following weekend. And then things turned worse again. Amy was admitted overnight for a grade IV allergic reaction to the drug. She stayed off the drug for two weeks to let her body heal, and then started on a lower dose.

Our summer was full of activities, which is par for the course with three children. Amy attended her high school reunion, while I stayed home with our kids. At the event, Amy started talking to her old boyfriend from high school and college, who then made the connection to Amy and her blog. He said, "I didn't follow your little Internet cancer adventure thing, but I'm so glad you beat that." That made her so angry that she graciously maneuvered an exit and got away to scream. She called me to share the experience. If I had been there with her, I probably would have punched him. Actually, I know I would have. I was so shocked and horrified that someone could say something so wrong. He was my fraternity brother and someone we both knew well, yet he still said something so crass.

As we were talking, Amy said, "Cancer is not an adventure. It's a nightmare for us, our family, and all the friends openhearted enough to get involved. Cancer is losing old friends who can't handle it, and my body disappointing me despite my ironclad desire to beat this thing. Cancer is pain, nausea, vomiting, hair loss, itching, fevers, chills, exhaustion, having parts removed and implanted, memory problems, and trying to miss as little as possible of what's left of my life. Cancer is waiting, waiting, and more waiting. It is worrying about our children, about whether I have seen my last sunrise. It is about acceptance. I have released my dreams of our retirement together and watching our kids graduate like balloons into the sky and watched them float away. It is too painful to cling to them, even though I have no guarantee of living that long without cancer." It was so hard to imagine how she was feeling in that moment as I sat thousands of miles away. She came home the next day.

At Amy's appointment with her oncologist in September, he recommended that she stop taking the Zelboraf and start the immunotherapy drug, called Yervoy. He scheduled her first infusion for October 1. She had two infusions and then on October 30, we heard some really tough news. Two brain tumors showed up on her scans. One had showed up on the scans in April, and the Zelboraf had shrunk it to nothing. Now it was back and six millimeters in size, and the other one was four millimeters, another low blow to this roller coaster ride that was our life. She told me she had said a prayer before going to pick up our kids from school that God bring her a rainbow and provide some guidance on how to accept this news. When she left to take our daughter to soccer practice, she had another rainbow experience. When she returned and walked in the door, she said, "Did you see the rainbow? I know what you are thinking; I'm crazy because it's not raining. When we topped the hill coming down our street just now, it was way up in the sky, right over our house." Our daughter proceeded to corroborate the story and said they had seen the rest of the rainbow on the way to soccer practice.

These experiences with the rainbows gave Amy comfort and injected her with hope and strength to endure more treatments. She started again on the Zelboraf to try to shrink her heart tumor, which had grown by this point. She was able to finish the four infusions of Yervoy. In early December, she also had the SRS radiation, which is a focused form of high-dose radiation that zapped the tumors in her brain and killed them. She was unable to drive for three months after the procedure. We hired someone to help with shuttling our kids to and from school and their various activities. We celebrated the 2012 Christmas and New Year's holidays mostly at home, and then were able to get away to Colorado for a snow skiing trip with our children.

We enjoyed another six months of living our life in an as normal state as possible and then heard tough news again. Amy's heart tumor had grown rapidly. Up to this point, the doctor had told us that surgery really wasn't an option, as it was too risky. We were in the hospital for scans when the cardiac surgeon came in the room. He said a surgery like this had never been done, but he thought he could do it. There were risks that she wouldn't survive the surgery. Then he said, in a matter-of-fact tone, "If she doesn't have the surgery, she will probably never leave the hospital." After he left, it took us only a minute to agree that she should have the surgery.

Amy had the heart surgery in August. It felt like I was watching paint dry as I sat there waiting, looking at the doors as they opened, hoping to see Amy's surgeon walk out with an update. Knowing how risky this surgery was, my fear kept trying to take over my mind. The procedure seemed to drag on and on. One of the moms from our daughter's soccer team was the doctor in charge of the equipment that kept Amy's blood flowing while her heart was stopped. It was comforting to me to know that she was in there with Amy during the entire procedure. I breathed a sigh of relief when the surgeon came into the waiting room to announce that the surgery had been a success, and I would be able to see her soon. While Amy believed the surgery was important, her recovery was long and painful. On her worst days, she would say it was worth it, though. That surgery gave us one more Halloween with the kids, one more Thanksgiving with our families, and one more Christmas.

One weekend in November, I was at a cars and coffee event with my sons, walking around and checking out the cars. I met a fellow Porsche owner, and we started talking about our lives. Somehow the subject of Amy came up, and I told him what was going on with her. He asked if I had ever heard of Gilda's Club and said his dad was a counselor there. I thanked him for the advice and met his dad for coffee a week later. He had lost his wife to cancer and raised his three children on his own. He asked a lot of questions about us, our plans, and how our kids were coping. He gave me some confidence that we had been doing all the right things to prepare for the inevitable.

After Christmas, we had planned a quick family vacation to Key West. The morning we were supposed to fly out, Amy was very sick and was shaking all over. I tried to tell her there was no way she could travel like this. She gritted her teeth, gave me that look I knew all too well when her mind was made up, and said "I. Am. Going." We were able to enjoy Key West despite Amy's deteriorating health. It was helpful to change our scenery to distract us from what we were facing, and to create some lasting family memories.

As we made it through January, it felt like her time was getting closer. The topic of hospice came up as we entered February. The original plan was to have someone from hospice come to the house once a day to check on her. Amy didn't want to pass away at home—she thought that would be harder on the kids. So the new plan was for the hospice nurse to tell us when she thought it was time for us to come in. We would then move Amy to the hospice residence hall.

We had our initial meeting with hospice at our house on February 19, 2014, and they explained how the process worked and what to expect. I remember sitting on the couch, holding Amy's hand as we planned for the end. It seemed so surreal that this was really happening. I thought we'd have a couple more weeks together, maybe a month. The nurse called me a few hours after they left our house and said "Alan, based on what I observed in Amy's first visit, we feel like she needs to come in now and not wait." I was in the car when they called, and I remember pulling into a parking lot and just sobbing. A waterfall of tears poured down my cheeks as I sorted out the reality of what she had just said. After fighting for four years, her time to leave was near. I gathered my wits about me and headed home to tell Amy, one of the hardest and most gut-wrenching things I have ever done in my life. She was surprisingly calm and at peace about it. We packed a small bag, she hugged our kids and our dog Pepper, and she told the kids they could come see her tomorrow as we left.

Our experience with hospice was supportive and compassionate. The spiritual counselor explained what we might experience as her time to leave drew near—that Amy might see people or hear things not visible or audible to the average human. I didn't quite believe the counselor. Sure enough, mid-afternoon the day before she died, Amy said, "Hey, Alan, I hear singing. Do you hear that? I think it must be the sisters from the Catholic school." I didn't hear anything. Amy had a special connection with the sisters and could hear them, although our location was about four miles away. Amy greeted many friends and family in her last days and died on February 22 surrounded by love.

Amy died around ten at night with her mom and me by her side, holding her hands. Going home and telling the kids she was gone was another gut-wrenching conversation that broke me to my core. They would no longer have a mom around to help them, fuss at them, and share memories with. While we'd had warning that this day was coming, there is nothing that could have prepared me or my children for such a deep loss of the heart. Amy's mom spent the night at our house that night, and I think we finally went to bed around one o'clock. I don't think I slept a lot that night, but I was able to rouse myself out of bed around seven when I heard Amy's mom in the kitchen.

The sun was rising and shining through our bedroom window. As I walked toward the kitchen, I noticed a bright rainbow prism of light coming through the window and hitting the floor. I went and grabbed Amy's mom and showed her so she wouldn't think I was crazy. The rainbow prism of light felt like such a clear message from Amy saying that she had made it to the other side and was okay. It was deeply comforting in the midst of my grief of losing her, and it felt like our connection would remain strong. A few weeks later, when I was talking to the principal at my kids' Catholic school, he told me that the sisters had in fact been singing and praying for Amy and our family at the time when Amy said she heard them, the day before she died.

Amy and I dated for six years and were married for twenty years. The helpful part of our cancer experience is we had time, time to spend together, to say what we wanted to say, and to plan. Amy wrote letters to each of our kids and to me, and she planned her entire funeral. Her direct orders were: "No fucking peace lilies." Amy told me at the beginning of her cancer experience that she needed me to be her rock. She used to tease me about always being such an optimist and always being positive, but now she needed that from me. She battled to keep from slipping into "deep dark places" as she called them, so we didn't cry a lot around each other. We didn't talk about her odds of surviving or about the end, other than her planning her funeral. There were times when it couldn't be helped, but she didn't want to dwell on the bad things. She wanted our life, and our kids' lives, to be as "normal" as possible.

I believe that every family is different, and every kid is different. For us, we thought we needed to be open and honest with our kids about what was happening. We didn't want to scare them, but it seemed pointless to pretend this wasn't happening as it unfolded in our daily lives. We didn't talk about survival chances or surgery risks, but each time something new emerged that we needed to face, we tried to tell them what the doctors would do, how it would make Mom feel, and what she'd look like when she came home, whether with bandages, drains, or oxygen tanks. For our kids, I think this approach helped lessen the impact of the experience.

When Amy was first diagnosed with cancer, we were reluctant to accept help from people. We had both always been very independent and didn't feel like we needed meals or someone to pick up our kids from school or activities. What we learned pretty quickly is that we really did need help. Amy needed to rest, and cooking, cleaning, and driving became exhausting for her. We also recognized that people really wanted to do something, anything that we needed to help us. I imagine that helping us was in part a way to process their feelings of powerlessness over what we were going through. Although they had no control over our story, they could step in and lessen the impact of our difficult experience. Our kids' school and our church were amazing sources of support and strength. I remember one night we were all sitting at home before one of Amy's surgeries. I noticed something outside the window and got up to take a look.

There were probably a hundred or more people gathered in our front yard with candles to sing and pray together for Amy.

After Amy died, the young woman I had hired to help with the kids got a great job and moved on. My daughter was away at a travel soccer tournament while I was interviewing for a nanny. She called me and asked, "Dad, what are you looking for in a nanny? I would rather you not hire someone who might be mistaken for my mom. That would be weird." I was relieved to have her input and hired a twenty-one-year-old woman.

While Amy's faith grew deeper during this trying time, my experience was the opposite. The outpouring of love and support from friends and family was invaluable and got us through such a tough time. I really appreciated people helping us so selflessly. I grew disenchanted with the dogma of the Catholic religion during the experience, though, in part following a conversation with the principal of my younger son's Catholic school. We were sitting in her office one day when she told me that God wants us to suffer in order for us to get closer to Him. That really turned me off. I remain a spiritual person, but I have turned away from the Catholic Church.

The woman from Arkansas whom we met in Houston with stage IV cancer is still living. That is a great testament to defying the numbers. The numbers are averages, and none of us are average. I still keep in touch with this couple, and we see each other when we travel to Knoxville to watch University of Tennessee football games.

When I think back to right after Amy died, I remember feeling that if the kids were doing okay, then I was okay. My friend's dad encouraged me to come to a grief support group at Gilda's Club one night. I was reluctant to go, but I eventually gave in. I actually got more out of it than I expected. A year or so later, Gilda's Club started another group called "No Time to Grieve." It was a grief support group specifically for people like me who had lost a spouse to cancer and were raising kids alone. This group became like a family to me. Finally, I had people who could *truly* relate to what I was going through.

It has now been over five years since Amy has passed. Our kids went through some hard times; well, actually, we all did. I believe that our kids watching their mom battle cancer the way they did has shaped them in some positive ways. They don't dwell on the little, petty things that some of their peers get so upset about. It has given them a more mature perspective on life. I'm certainly closer to the three of them now than I ever was before. I've probably overindulged a bit with them at times, such as the first Christmas without Amy, but I guess that's just me trying to make up for their shitty childhoods. We have had a lot of fun and enjoyed some great trips together. We still talk about Amy frequently and laugh about the funny things she used to do. It's important for me to keep her memory alive with them, especially my youngest son who was only seven when she died. On Amy's birthday we always get her a cake, as she *loved* birthday cake, and then we watch old home movies. It's always a bit of a shock to hear her voice and laughter again after so long.

We still see rainbows at odd times. I've seen them in relatively clear skies on our wedding anniversary or on birthdays. And when our son Parker made his First Holy Communion a couple months after she passed away, the cathedral was full of rainbows of light as he walked down the aisle toward the altar. Whenever the kids and I see one now, it feels like Amy saying hello and reminding us that she loves and watches over us.

Advice for Others

How we supported each other
- We really maximized time to talk and created lifelong memories when possible.
- We were transparent with our children from the start.
- We tried to really take advantage of those times when Amy was feeling good and do fun things.
- We loved to travel and didn't let cancer get in the way of taking trips with our children.

- If there is a silver lining in our cancer experience, it is that it gave us some time to plan and talk before the end.
- The letters that Amy wrote us, and her blog, are the gifts that I think we all cherish the most.
- Being open with our kids enabled us to have them go to counseling prior to the end to help them prepare.

How others supported us
- We were well supported over the four years by friends, family, and our community with countless meals, errand running, and shuttling our children to and from school and activities.
- We felt the bottomless prayers from our family, friends, and community as we endured each step.
- Members of the church came to sing and pray for Amy before her surgeries.

Helpful tips
- If you are facing a cancer diagnosis or know someone who is, use the time you have and don't leave anything left unsaid.
- When you face hard times, surrender and let people help; it helps both of you.
- If you are a spouse of someone who has cancer, get counseling, and if you have children, offer counseling to them as well.

KRISTI'S STORY

———— • ● • ————

G reg and I married in 2006, both bringing children from previous marriages to our new family. In the early part of 2015,
I remember Greg having a red spot on his chest that looked like
an infected hair follicle. He and I talked about it, and he decided
to get it checked out. He went to an urgent care clinic, thinking
it was nothing. The doctor examined him and said, "Greg, I don't
think this is anything to be concerned about. Looks like it might
be fatty tissue." Greg was an avid golfer, golfing most days as we
lived on a golf course. Our busy lives took over and a few months
passed. The spot was still there. His golf shirts would rub on the
spot, and it kept bothering him, which led him to make an appointment with a dermatologist. He went to the appointment alone in
mid-June 2015, as we didn't think it was anything to be worried
about. The dermatologist examined him and said, "It looks like
it's just a cyst, probably nothing to worry about, although it does
appear inflamed. It may be infected, so let's start you on antibiotics
to see if it gets better, and then we can talk about what to do next.
I'll send the prescription to your pharmacy. Let's have you come
back in a month."

In mid-July, when the spot was still there, Greg returned to
the dermatologist. The spot seemed to be getting more inflamed

despite the antibiotics. After examining it, the doctor decided to remove the cyst and send it to the lab for evaluation. After he removed it, he commented that it wasn't a normal cyst—it "had a tail on it," which had us thinking it might be cancer, as we both worked in healthcare. He said it would take a couple of weeks to get the results. While we were starting to think it might be skin cancer, we thought it was treatable and not something to worry about.

At the end of July, Greg heard from the dermatologist who said, "Greg, the pathology came back a little odd. It's pretty common to get a consult on tissue samples. I would like to send it off to a specialist in Ohio, just to make sure. I think it will probably take a couple of weeks to get the results back, and I'll give you a call." When Greg and I sat down for dinner that evening, he told me what the doctor said. Even though the doctor said it was standard protocol to get a second opinion, both Greg and I started to wonder what it might be. I still wasn't super worried. Greg had lived in Phoenix and spent several days a week outside playing golf for seventeen years. He was fair skinned, and dermatologists in the past had said if he was going to get skin cancer, it would show up somewhere other than on the exposed skin. From what the doctor had said in the past, the most sensitive parts of your skin are where cancer typically comes up to the surface, versus the hardened skin that has been exposed to the sun. Greg's spot was on his chest, covered by his shirt.

On August 12, I was traveling for work in North Carolina and was at the airport heading home, traveling with a coworker. Just then, my phone rang, and it was Greg. "Hey, my doctor just called and asked me to come into the office later today to discuss the results." It was a Wednesday, which was the doctor's normal day to do surgery, not to see patients in the office. It gave me pause to think he was calling and wanted to meet on a day without office hours. Greg made plans to be at the office during my layover in Charlotte so I could join in by phone. I tried to distract myself during the flight, although we were still thinking he was going to say Greg had skin cancer. I landed in Charlotte and called Greg, who was with the dermatologist. The doctor looked at him and said, in a very matter-of-fact way, "You've got cancer, Greg. It's small cell lung cancer that has grown through the chest wall."

As the words permeated my mind, I asked, speaking from a place of disbelief, "How can you possibly tell that it is small cell lung cancer from a spot on his chest?"

He replied, "We can tell by the type of cells. It's stage IV, because the cyst I removed was a secondary site. You need to get into see your primary care physician as soon as possible." I was stunned and speechless. He again recommended getting an appointment quickly with Greg's primary care physician, and I hung up.

As tears started streaming down my cheeks, Greg called me. I felt horrible not being there with him as he sorted out the shocking diagnosis he had just heard. The only thing I could do was to take action. We made a plan and hung up. I was struggling with how he must be feeling, hearing that news and being alone. I called his doctor's office and made an appointment for X-rays for the next morning. I worked for a large healthcare company and knew the president of the cancer division. After making the appointment, I also left a message for the president asking her for advice on what to do next. By the time I landed in Nashville, I had a message from her. She said she would be happy to help connect us to clinical trials and most important, to get into see an oncologist quickly. She had made an appointment for Greg for Friday at 7:30 in the morning. When I arrived home, I wrapped my arms around Greg as we both cried and shared our feelings, horribly in shock and trying to make sense of it all. Then I said, "We are going to fight this together." The rest of the night was a blur, due to the stress of the situation and the news we were still sorting out.

The next morning, we showed up for the doctor's appointment. After he examined Greg, he sent him for X-rays. The doctor came back in quickly and said that he could see several tumors in both of his lungs. He said, "It is really important that you see somebody soon and start treatment." I said we had an appointment with an oncologist already scheduled for the next morning. He offered to help us however he could, and we left, still in a place of bewilderment and disbelief. That night, we asked Greg's son to come to the house and called my daughter by phone, as she was away at college. His son was twenty-nine at the time, and my daughter was twenty, ready to start her senior year of her undergraduate program. There was no good way to start the conversation. I decided to be transparent and straightforward and told them what we had heard. I watched as our new reality settled into our children's hearts and tears started streaming down their faces. We hugged and cried together, then I said, "We have the right doctors, and we are going to get through this together."

At 7:30 on Friday, we arrived early for Greg's oncology appointment, were met by the chief medical officer, and were fast tracked back to the office of the head of clinical trials. She said there was one option for a notch inhibitor trial that we could try, but no full-blown drug trials for small cell. She offered to keep us posted if that changed. Then we met with the oncologist, who said it would be good to start with chemotherapy, which was standard and the only available treatment for small cell lung cancer. The oncologist scheduled a series of scans for the following Monday morning, the 17th. We left with more information and somewhat of a plan. The weekend felt really long as I moved around mostly in a fog, overwhelmed and distressed. Through many conversations over the weekend, Greg and I bonded strongly, determined to fight the cancer together. My daughter flew home from college on Saturday, in order to be with us as we collectively learned about and considered our next steps. I realized by the end of the weekend how our focus had shifted, and everything else that we had been worrying about fell away. We became ultra-focused on getting Greg the treatment he needed and leveraging whatever relationships we had to make it happen quickly.

On Monday morning, Greg and I drove to the imaging center for the scans. Greg's son and my daughter met us there.

Greg endured a CT scan, bone scan, MRI, and PET scan, which spanned several hours. The technician said they would send the results to the doctor, and she would call us to discuss them. We left the imaging center and went to eat barbecue for lunch at one of our favorite local restaurants. We tried to keep the conversation light over lunch and put aside what we were facing for a few minutes. After lunch, as we were driving home on I65, the oncologist's office called and said, "Greg, we need you to come back to your oncologist's office immediately. We found seven lesions in your brain, and your brain is swollen." The doctor went on to say how shocked she was that he wasn't experiencing headaches, having seizures, or feeling a serious imbalance. His brain was so swollen that it was pushed off to one side of his head.

Greg said, "No, I feel fine. I need to get home and play golf."

The doctor replied, "We have to get what is going on in your brain under control. I think you should get radiation this afternoon, although I would like to get the radiation oncologist's opinion first. We'll quickly draw some blood while you are here, and then send you to his office. They are waiting for you."

While Greg had left the exam room to get his blood drawn, I asked the doctor what we should be thinking about or expecting here. She said, "I don't like to put a time frame on people's lives because everyone is different. Given his brain condition and the advanced nature of his cancer, his time left is very short, maybe eight weeks." I swallowed so deeply you could probably have heard the gulp down the hall. I decided not to tell Greg what she had said.

When Greg came back, he announced, "I don't want to know how long I have. This is my story. I'm going to live my story my way." It was sobering to hear him say these words, as I was still processing what I had heard from the doctor. As we were walking to the radiation oncologist's office, I assured him that we would walk this path together, however long it was. We were rushed back to the exam room quickly.

The doctor came in, introduced himself, and said, "Greg, you actually have lesions in all four quadrants of your brain. I want to take time to build a detailed plan for your radiation as it will be a whole-brain radiation, impacting every aspect, including short term memory and normal daily functions. My goal is to try to preserve your cognitive ability to the greatest degree possible." The doctor ordered steroids to reduce Greg's brain swelling. We learned that in addition to immediately starting his chemotherapy regimen of Carboplatin and Etoposide, which required six three-week cycles, the only way to treat the extensive cancer at this stage was to do radiation at the same time, due to the pervasive nature of the tumors. We left and headed back home, hoping that the waiting would not be long. Greg continued playing golf almost daily, not demonstrating any visible signs that he was sick with late-stage cancer. For me, the waiting was debilitating. I found myself losing track of what I was doing some days, as my mind would wander forward to what might happen next. I am a planner, and without a plan, I felt like each day was moving by in slow motion. Finally, two weeks later, we had a plan for whole-brain radiation.

Before Greg's diagnosis, we had been planning a full remodel of our 6,200-square-foot home on the golf course that we had purchased in 2010. We were in the process of securing financing, hiring a builder, and hiring a decorator when we learned of Greg's condition. The week after his diagnosis was when we secured all three of these components. I was not sure going through a remodel with a husband who had just been diagnosed with stage IV cancer was a good idea, and I decided to let Greg make this call. I said, "Honey, we now have all of the necessary pieces in place to move forward with the remodel. Do you want to go through with it and move out or stop the remodel and stay in the house? I am good with whatever you want."

He said it gave him hope to go through with the remodel, as it provided him something positive to focus on, something to look forward to in our future. I smiled and said, "Okay, we'll go forward. So you know that means we'll have to move into an apartment. Would you prefer to be in your normal environment while you are going through treatment or are you comfortable with being someplace new?" Greg decided that being in a smaller space might actually be better, as I worked long hours and traveled, leaving him home alone for long periods. In that moment, we both believed that he would beat this cancer. Once we made the decision to move forward with the remodel, everything started changing. We had to move everything out of the house into a two-bedroom apartment near my office.

Treatment Experience

Greg started his whole-brain radiation two weeks after his diagnosis at the end of August. He would go in every weekday for three weeks and a total of fifteen treatments. He started chemotherapy infusions the same week. I drove him most days, although he would sometimes drive himself. To prepare for the radiation, they made a mask. During the treatment, the technician would lock him down to the table so his head wouldn't move. The treatments would take about thirty minutes. He experienced some forgetfulness and would see colored lights, beams of light sometimes. The doctor was trying to preserve his cognitive ability, although during the treatments his cognitive functioning got worse. He still drove. What I still think about is that Greg did not experience any glaring or visibly noticeable symptoms. He endured both radiation and chemotherapy at the same time due to the advanced nature of his cancer. Because he was so healthy and strong, the doctor believed he could handle it.

While he was getting the radiation treatment for his brain, the white matter grew in his brain, and he became very forgetful. I would find pieces of paper with his name, phone number and address on it in his pockets and on pads of paper around the house.

One day he said we needed to pick up his dry cleaning which he had dropped off. We went together one afternoon to our regular dry cleaner near our apartment and found they didn't have his clothes. He was getting short-tempered and angry with the woman behind the counter when she said she didn't have our laundry. Greg didn't believe her and demanded to go in the back to look for his clothes. While he was in the back, I walked home a block away, found the dry-cleaning slip, and returned with it. She looked it and said, "That is not from our store." When Greg realized he was wrong, he started apologizing for getting so angry. He felt awful. We thanked them and went to get in the car.

I asked, "Do you know where you took the dry cleaning?"

A blank stare filled Greg's face. "I have no idea," he said. The receipt didn't have a name on it, just a phone number. I called the number and found out where they were located. It was a dry cleaner store near our house. We drove over to get the dry cleaning together. That night when we were back at home, I was concerned about his memory and ordered a device to track his car. He was very stubborn and refused to stop driving, reiterating to me that he was fine. With all he was facing, the last thing I wanted to do was take his freedom away. He continued to play golf most days. Some days, he was only able to play nine holes. From the day Greg was diagnosed, he couldn't work anymore, so golf is how he filled his days. He always thought he would go back to work, although after he started treatment, he could no longer process things sequentially.

We met another individual named Ronn, who had been diagnosed with lung cancer and was in treatment at the time Greg started his treatment. Ronn's story appears in another chapter in this book. We were introduced to him through a friend and saw him on one of Greg's first treatments. He ended up becoming a dear friend and a huge support to Greg and me as we walked Greg's treatment path and endured the physical and emotional challenges we faced. Greg handled both the chemotherapy and radiation treatments well, with minimal side effects. He was more tired than usual. By the middle of December, his doctor reported that the tumors had shrunk significantly; the treatment had been extremely effective. Some of the tumors were no longer visible. She announced, "Let's give you some time off, say three months, and see what happens." We enjoyed the holidays, celebrating the progress of Greg's treatment and working on our remodel. During this time, we met with an attorney and established living wills, as well as general and healthcare powers of attorney. We also made a list of all of Greg's personal possessions, noting where he wanted things to go should he die. We then took all those items and locked them away in the safe. With the comfort of these discussions behind us, we were able to go back to our lives and focus on living.

Greg returned to his doctor on January 5 for a checkup and scans. Our balloons of hope were deflated when we learned his cancer was growing again and he needed some type of treatment. He had already taken all the chemotherapy his body would handle. Fortunately, we were told at that point, "There is a clinical trial for non-small cell lung cancer that was just approved for use in small cell lung cancer patients on December 22nd. It is a two-armed trial of Opdivo and Yervoy. You could get one of the drugs or randomize to the study group to receive both drugs. If you had presented two weeks ago, we would not have been able to offer it to you." We looked at each other, feeling the hand of God working through the system and creating options.

Greg's doctor recommended he enroll in the trial, and he did. Greg was chosen to receive both drugs, which made the doctor and us very happy. The trial proved to be helpful, although he did experience some of the side effects they had warned us might be possible, including blood clots in his lung that they treated with steroids. Overall, he was managing well and several months went by. My daughter and I had planned a trip to Washington DC for the weekend to celebrate her twenty-first birthday, which was on May 13, 2016. That morning before we left, Greg had an appointment for labs. The results came back showing elevated liver enzymes, indicating he was experiencing treatment related hepatitis, which required hospitalization because of his weakened immune system. We went home, packed his bag, and checked him into the hospital. He kept begging us to take him home so he could play golf. He said he felt fine and was not happy about having to be admitted. My daughter and I cancelled our trip and decided to go to a nice steak place to celebrate that night. There we were, all dressed up, in lovely dresses and fancy shoes, sitting next to each other and weeping at the table. We were quite a sight for others around us to see in the restaurant. The doctors were quickly able to get the inflammation in Greg's liver under control, and he was able to return home to his regular routine within a couple of days.

Greg was a sports fan and had places and events he had always wanted to visit but hadn't had the chance to, including seeing the Chicago Cubs play at Wrigley Field. I decided to try to get him to a game before the end of the season and began looking for tickets. That sports trip took on a life of its own. Before I knew it, I had scheduled an entire week for us to travel, including a visit to the Louisville Slugger museum and factory, Oktoberfest in Chicago, the final Cubs game at Wrigley Field, a Packers game at Lambeau Field, a night in Cincinnati to celebrate my fiftieth birthday, and tickets to a Pittsburgh Steelers game from the fifty-yard line. I offered to take him to a University of Tennessee football game, but Greg was worn out and ready to go home.

The stress of keeping up with the remodel and supporting Greg through his treatments, along with my job responsibilities, was pushing me close to my breaking point. Greg was struggling more with memory and decision-making issues, which required me to take on management of the remodel project, along with everything else. One morning, I brought up the conversation with Greg. "Hey, can we talk about the house remodel? I just want to talk through it with you. My sense is it will take you a while to regain your strength. It is just becoming too much for me to manage given our situation. I am not giving up on you at all; I just want to enjoy life more with you rather than being focused on the remodel. What do you think?"

He did not take the conversation well, but after giving it more thought agreed that we needed a different plan. We decided to sell the house and buy a townhouse. As the dry wall was finished in our home, we put further work on hold and were able to find a buyer. Greg and I looked around the area for a neighborhood and a townhouse layout that would accommodate his increasing fatigue. It was also extremely important to him that we find a place that would be safe and secure for me to live in alone, should something happen to him. We found a gated neighborhood and a unit that had a lovely fenced-in courtyard where we thought we could enjoy the outdoor sitting area together. We were able to schedule closing on both properties for August 31st.

After the fact, I can see some things that were signs that something was off, although we didn't pay enough attention. When Greg tried to wakeboard behind a ski boat once, he had trouble balancing and couldn't stand up. It was extremely frustrating for him, but he simply didn't have the strength or balance required. He thought it was because of his one knee, which was extremely arthritic, and had planned to have surgery on in December of 2016. He was also having trouble lying flat in bed and getting comfortable, so we bought him a new bed to allow him to elevate his head.

On August 23rd, 2016, Greg went in for his regularly scheduled scans and lab work. Greg had been more lethargic the past week or so, and I sensed something wasn't right. I asked him about it, but he continued to say he thought he was fine and that maybe the summer heat was getting to him. When we met with the oncologist to get his scan and lab results, to our great surprise we were told, "Your tumors are gone." It was very exciting news for all of us. He was high fiving the doctor. Since Greg had just had his blood drawn, those lab results were not yet available. I told the doctor in front of Greg that I really believed something wasn't right.

In spite of my concerns, we needed to celebrate the great news we had received that day and did so by going out to dinner with dear friends at one of our favorite restaurants. Greg was elated that evening but noticeably fatigued, which caused all of us but Greg to be concerned. One friend having dinner with us that evening is a registered nurse. She commented to me privately that Greg did not look well, and I mentioned that the day's lab work was not back yet when we met with the doctor. When the lab results came in, they got filed without being reviewed. Five days later, Greg was much worse; he slept a lot and his urine was dark, the color of root beer. I called the doctor a couple of times to report that Greg's color didn't look good and that he was lethargic. She finally said to bring him in to hospital. He was hospitalized again on August 31, 2016. We closed on both the townhouse and our house on that same day, from Greg's hospital room.

The doctor motioned for me to come out in the hallway when we were finished and said, "I thought the reason you were being so negative was because you didn't want to allow yourself the positive moment, thinking of the big picture and what might be." I told her that while Greg was always positive and wanted things to be good, I felt in my gut that something wasn't adding up. I really wanted to be happy for him, although I needed to speak up. The doctor said that Greg had autoimmune hepatitis, as he'd had previously, and that his liver was failing. She tried everything and nothing worked. He was hospitalized for six days. He had been unable to rest well for days, although it seemed that all he had done was sleep. She gave him some heavy-duty drugs, and he slept for a day and a half. Because his liver was not working, it was unable to flush the drugs through his body, so the effects were much stronger. When he was in the hospital, I would go home overnight. When I would leave, Greg would cry and beg me to take him home. It tore my heart out to say good-bye every night as tears rolled down his face. As I think back to this time in Greg's last few days, my one regret is that I didn't sleep with him in the hospital at night. Over the course of the year, we had each said everything we wanted to say to the other, so it was more about just being present with him.

After six days in the hospital, the doctor discharged him home and arranged for hospice to come to our house. As Greg was being wheeled out to the car after being discharged, we happened to see Ronn leaving the hospital from a meeting. Ronn hugged Greg and "loaded" him into the car, a touching moment of connection and compassion. While there are many great stories of hospice experiences, our experience was not good. The hospice nurse was very kind and supportive but was less willing than I would have expected to have frank discussions. As Greg's condition deteriorated, I was surprised that the nurse kept saying he had several weeks left. I called Greg's oncologist and described what I was seeing and how I was getting conflicting messages from the hospice nurse. This experience challenged me to manage day to day effectively, as I was unsure of the timing and what we needed to be doing. While this nurse may have thought she was being helpful, it felt unfair for her to assume I was not able to handle the truth.

Greg's condition deteriorated rapidly in his last few days. The doctor tried steroids, antirejection drugs used with liver transplants, and finally some horrible medicine that smelled and tasted awful. Greg looked at me one morning and said, "I've had enough. I don't want to take this medicine anymore." I called the doctor and told her what he had said.

She said, "Does he realize if he doesn't take it, what he is choosing?" Greg could hear the conversation and smiled at me, nodding yes, as he had accepted his fate. Throughout Greg's illness, we had talked as a family with him about supporting whatever choices he made regarding receiving or refusing treatment at any point. We assured him it was a decision only he could make for himself, and we would be supportive of whatever he chose. It was hard to face the stark reality of Greg's decision, knowing the inevitable end was now likely near. He accepted his situation, and we had to as well.

While Greg was still able, we did meaningful things such as going out for pizza with friends and attending a baseball game for a friend's child, enabling Greg to visit with umpire friends. On his final trip out of the house, we took him for a pedicure, and to the country club we belonged to so he could visit with all of his golfing buddies for the afternoon and say good-bye. We lived in a two-bedroom apartment and had welcomed our family to be with us during these last days. Greg's sister and brother-in-law, his son, and my daughter all slept at our apartment. Our best friends, a couple that we vacationed and spent a lot of time with, also spent many days and evenings with us.

Given what he was facing, Greg decided he wanted all of his friends and family to come over and say good-bye. We hosted hundreds of loved ones over the course of five days. From an observer's point of view, it felt like he was holding court, as royalty does, from ten to six daily. He would tell funny stories and break out laughing. In the midst of the heart-wrenching reality that he had only days to live, he chose to fill them with love and joy and had the best time he could. Friends would come and laugh with him, hug him, and say good-bye, all the while doing a pretty good job of holding in their emotions. Then I would walk out with them one by one into the hallway to thank them for coming and for being so supportive to our family. That is when their emotions would become visible with tears pouring down their cheeks and I found myself comforting others for the loss they were experiencing. It was a surreal experience that I felt rather like a third party to. While Greg was home on hospice, I hired a male caregiver who was able to help with Greg's personal care and lift him in and out of the tub, wheelchair, and car. This helped allow me to try to maintain a bit of our relationship as husband and wife and to physically protect me from injury.

We were asleep in our bed at 3:30 on Saturday morning when Greg woke me up and wanted to plan his celebration of life. He asked my daughter to come in. He had obviously put a lot of thought into it and was excited to share his plans with us. He started with dessert, his favorite meal, and worked back from there. He wanted everyone to wear something bright, in their favorite color. He wanted people to hear music, laugh, tell stories, and have good memories of him, not to cry and be put through the emotional torture of a funeral. He had also known he wanted to be cremated and his ashes spread in New Hope in Mount Eagle, where the lakes meet. Greg had always loved Boyz II Men. I had bought tickets to their concert for the weekend before he died, but he was too weak to get out of bed to attend. His son created a playlist of Boyz II Men songs, and we played them for Greg that night as he lay in bed with his eyes closed. During a brief coherent period the next day, he told loved ones about how we had been to the concert and how much he enjoyed it. The last two days, he mostly slept. We stopped allowing visitors at this point. He said his last words to me, "I love you."

He died at 2:30 am on Tuesday, September 14, 2016. He lived thirteen full months from the day of his diagnosis, eleven more than the doctor had told me. He ended up dying of liver failure, which was a side effect of the immunotherapy. He was tumor free. The same people Greg wanted with him in his final few days of life joined us to scatter his ashes from a pontoon boat on October 16, right where he had requested.

"I can be one out of one," is what Greg would say, meaning his outcome of treatment can be different than anyone who had experienced a similar cancer situation before. "Every experience and body is different. If I don't make it through this, my hope is to help someone else. If the doctors can learn something, it will all be worth it." Doctors said there was no rational explanation as to how he was able to do all that he did. We traveled. He played golf. He wanted them to harvest all his organs and study anything they could. The doctor said while they can create drugs, they don't have the resources to study organs and learn from the experience. He was a rare blood donor with a strange antibody. There is no explanation other than God and his positive attitude.

I now live alone with no pets. As I reflect back, I am grateful that Greg and I got rid of 80 percent of what we owned. Some things that are missing I really don't miss. I have gone through two more layers and have started to realize how much our stuff owns us, including thoughts like *I have that. I am responsible for it. I can't just throw it away. That would not be responsible.*

The whole experience of Greg's diagnosis and death within a year has changed my perspective about life and how important it is to prioritize spending time on things that really matter. I think a lot about how Greg smoked for twenty years and never regretted it, although 100 percent of people who get small cell lung cancer have been smokers. I realized that having a bigger title and making more money was no longer meaningful as my focus. Nine months after Greg took his last breath; my position at work was eliminated, as the company I worked for was going in a different direction. I was still coping with the loss of Greg and now I'd lost my job. While I have always realized the value of my faith, my family, and my friends, experiencing these two deep losses within a nine-month period has led me to focus on who I am and to find joy in the little things. I am beyond grateful for the gift of welcoming each day. I am also delighted that Ronn, mentioned above, and I have developed such a bond through this experience that we have started a business together to provide support to patients. While I feel at peace now, I have struggled with it since Greg died. Greg and his father believed that there would be more people in heaven than we thought. I would love to know if that is true.

Advice for Others

How I supported myself
- I went to the gym at 4:30 every morning to work out and focus on myself.
- I developed a relationship with a therapist, who helped me work through the challenges.

- I kept working to give myself a break.
- After Greg died, I spent a lot of time hiking, enjoying nature and the outdoors.

How others supported me
- I was surrounded by family and friends.
- I accepted help from others, things like providing meals and taking Greg to treatments, and I became more willing to ask others for help.

Helpful tips
- If you are facing a cancer diagnosis or know someone who is, have the hard conversations early and be prepared for any outcome so you can enjoy each day.
- One of the nicest things someone can do for the family is to plan everything.
- Each of us has a story, and sometimes we don't know what the other is going through; I would recommend being more gracious with others and accepting of each person as they are.
- If you are a person who believes in God, learn to accept the path that unfolds each day; with time away from work, I have become more accepting of God's plan for my life in the past year.

Surprising experiences

In March of 2016, my daughter and I took a trip to Clearwater Beach, for her college spring break. Greg was still having treatments, and the house construction continued, so he suggested we take a break away from all we were dealing with and spend a few days at the beach. The morning after we arrived, I woke up early and went for a walk on the beach to watch the sunrise. I was listening to Christian music and was amazed as I looked around that I had the beach to myself. As I took each step, feeling the sand between my toes and watching the waves crashing a foot away, peace filled my heart. Suddenly, a vision of two women started to take shape in the distance. Within a moment, they were right next to me. One came and walked toward me near the water. She tapped me on the shoulder and said, "I can tell that you are really struggling with something. I can see it. I hope that you are not offended that I am sharing this with you."

I was stunned by her ability to read my thoughts and know where I was in my heart. She continued, "I need to tell you that things are going to be okay. I want you to be at peace with it. Just walk easy. Things will be okay. You have a beautiful aura around you." She had a warm smile, and light exuded from her body. I walked ten more steps, and with each step, the overwhelming feeling of emotion I felt in my heart expanded. I was sorting out what she had said in my mind, and tears started pouring out of my eyes. As I took a few more steps, I realized I hadn't asked the woman what she was talking about or how she knew. I was in my own little world. I looked up and the two women had disappeared. As I stood there, sorting out what had just happened, that the women had appeared out of nowhere and spoken to me in an omniscient way, knowing me intimately, and then disappeared as quickly as they appeared—I knew they had to be my guardian angels.

EPILOGUE

———•●•———

The process of writing this book has been enlightening and life-giving to me and now, I hope, to you. I believe that my own experience with my mom—who survived late-stage breast cancer while I was in college and died from colorectal cancer twenty years later—provided helpful exposure to the cancer journey with a loved one and honed a compassion and humility in me necessary to draw out the special stories captured in this book. Robyn and I reached out to people we knew asking for stories, and we easily found nineteen people willing to be vulnerable and share their very personal story with you, the reader. I remain humbled by the courage each person has shown to open up and share his or her innermost thoughts on a time in their life that was less than perfect. That is a tough act to uphold in our culture of perfection. I am also grateful for each person's willingness to relive the trauma that resurfaced as they shared the details of their story.

With the increasing incidence of cancer in our world, and close to 40 percent of us getting a cancer diagnosis in our lifetime, each of us will be touched in some way by this disease. Nearly one in two men and over one in three women will be diagnosed in their lifetime. As we walk this path ourselves or with a friend or loved one, know that advancements in cancer treatment are being made every day. It is helpful to research the latest treatments if you are facing a cancer diagnosis. One example is the Cancer Vaccine Institute. It was originally focused on vaccines that would prevent cancer from coming back and now is focused on preventing cancer. This institute is developing vaccines for breast, colon, ovarian, prostate, and lung cancers. To learn more, visit https://depts.washington.edu/tumorvac/home. Cancer treatment and surgery take an extreme toll on your body. Aaron and Meg Grunke founded the Survivor Fitness Foundation, an organization that empowers cancer survivors with the tools and training needed to fully recover health and wellness. To learn more, visit: https://survivorfitness.org/.

• • •

Dr. Scot Sedlacek was an oncologist in Denver who treated Robyn and several other patients in this book. He graciously agreed to share his perspective on the role of the doctor in the cancer journey and what he experienced before he retired last year. The following was adapted from an interview in 2018:

I had wanted to be a doctor since age five, as I come from a family of doctors, and my wife is a doctor. I practiced for thirty-five years and specialized in the most treatable type of cancer, breast cancer. Some of my patients stayed with me for over twenty years, and I developed friendships with them. As their doctor, it was tough when I saw patients who weren't managing the treatment well. These women carried a palpable worry with them, as if the weight of the world was on their shoulders. Every time one of my patients died, it took a piece of me. I chose the path of offering options and being supportive of my patients' decisions. Like the time when a patient stopped chemotherapy treatment because she didn't want to lose her hair. I respected that, although I didn't want her to die.

The three most important parts of my role as an oncologist while I was practicing were:

- Keeping up on the literature by reading journals and attending meetings and continuing medical education sessions. Being curious to learn about all aspects of the patient's situation and clinical details enabled me to recommend the right treatment for that patient.
- Being a cheerleader for my patient, telling them I wanted them to finish, and I needed them to be strong and push through to beat the cancer. I believe that the positive psychology of encouraging them, supporting them, and maintaining an inspirational tone makes a difference with patient outcomes.
- Being a friend as well. Being compassionate along the journey, especially when outcomes turn out differently than I thought.

I would be remiss if I didn't mention the role that faith played in my life. It was a pivotal part of my being able to practice in the breast cancer field for thirty-five years. The work I did was very satisfying, and my faith buoyed me many times when I saw tough outcomes. One of the common threads I saw with my patients was not feeling comfortable asking for help. I heard many times that women didn't want to inconvenience their friends. While I realize it may be hard for some to receive, I encouraged each patient to be vulnerable and let others in, let them help. We are all broken in some way, and community is how we survive and thrive in this journey called life.

• • •

Each chapter of this book includes advice for others based on the individual's personal experience. I have synthesized the common advice from each of the stories in this book below to give you a kind of cheat sheet to keep with you. May the following be a helpful guide along the cancer path.

- Every single cancer experience is unique: Be thoughtful about saying things like "I understand how you feel" or "I know what you are going through," even if you are a survivor.

- Make sure the family of the cancer patient has the support they need and a safe place to process their emotions.
- For someone who is newly diagnosed, interview other survivors and gather insights.
- Value your health and stay current on preventive screenings; seek care if you experience symptoms.
- Engage with your friend, acquaintance, or loved one when you learn of a diagnosis and acknowledge the situation—including saying you have no words if that is the case, or say, "I heard something about you that makes me sad or worried about you, you are in my thoughts and prayers;" know that withdrawing feels hurtful to the cancer patient.
- If you have not experienced a cancer diagnosis, don't say, "I understand what you are going through;" while well intended, it comes across as inauthentic.
- Learn how to advocate for yourself every single day, and learn how to trust yourself, that you know what you need.
- Keep a positive attitude; it's the key to staying focused on healing.
- Embrace emotions; it's okay to be vulnerable and cry.
- Encourage someone living with a cancer diagnosis to not let the cancer define them; add normal life activities back as soon as feasible.
- Food smells are challenging for many cancer patients—if you are cooking for one, keep the food very bland.
- Think about the comments you make when you see someone you think has cancer and try to be considerate of how it will be received.
- If you want to do something, set up a meal train and put in dietary restrictions; go buy household staples like toilet paper, paper towels, and laundry soap, all things people need, and then drop it off on the front porch.
- Don't sweat the small stuff; focus on the big picture.

- When you see someone who has a look about them that something is out of place, tell them they look great, that they have a great smile or something like that; don't be afraid to speak up and break the silence.
- Follow your gut—if doctors are not doing what you think they should, keep pushing for answers and keep asking questions.
- Know that the person with cancer is navigating life from a whole new perspective, learning new things about their body and the treatment every day.
- Cancer is a roller coaster ride: it is normal to cry and then start laughing ninety seconds later.
- Have the hard conversations early and be prepared for any outcome so you can enjoy each day.
- If you are a person who believes in God, learn to accept the path that unfolds each day and find the silver linings.

ACKNOWLEDGMENTS

———•—●—•———

The process of writing this book was divinely guided from the start. The idea came to me as I was praying for my friend Melissa—who had just been diagnosed with cancer. It was as if Jesus was talking to me directly, saying that I needed to stop working on the book I thought I was supposed to write and start this one. Shortly after this experience, I was having lunch with my dear friend Robyn and Jesus spoke again, saying I was to get Robyn's help. Robyn willingly stepped in and, between the two of us, we quickly found people who were comfortable sharing their personal stories in an effort to help others. Robyn brought a sense of comfort to all who participated, as she is a survivor herself. Thank you, Robyn, for helping make this book possible!

Writing this book consumed many waking hours of my nights and weekends, taking me away from my loved ones. I am deeply grateful for the countless hours of support from my children, family, and friends as I walked this path of writing my second book. I am also humbled beyond words for the following brave souls who chose to share their stories in order to help others: Melissa, Robyn, Helen, Ronn, Jennifer, Bill K., Dana, Bill G., Valerie, Dan, Peggy, Robert, Holly, Nikki, Kim, Gina, Tricia, Debi, Alan, and Kristi. Thank you for your patience as we worked through the details and brought your story to life on these pages. I appreciate each of you from the bottom of my heart!

I am also grateful for the expert advice and leadership of my publisher, Brooke Warner, and the She Writes Press team. Thank you for making this second publishing process smooth and hassle-free for me. I am also appreciative of my publicist Hannah and owner Julie of Books Forward, for guidance during the launch preparation and for leading the successful promotion and launch of this book.

I am honored that you have chosen to read this book. Thank you.

ABOUT THE AUTHOR:

Rebecca Whitehead Munn

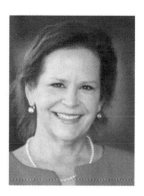

R ebecca is passionate about rethinking possible and brings intellectual humility to all of her endeavors, including several teaching roles at the master's level. Her passion in writing is to demystify taboo topics, such as cancer and death, and to inspire others to be courageous and learn about their loved ones' wishes, while creating life-long connections. Rebecca's award-winning debut memoir, *The Gift of Goodbye: A Story of Agape Love,* is her personal story of walking the End of Life path with her mother. She has been a featured Maria Shriver Architect of Change on surviving grief and shared her healing through yoga story at www. mindbodygreen.com. She holds a certification in the Foundations of Positive Psychology from University of Pennsylvania, is a certified End of Life Doula, and a Nashville Healthcare Council Fellow.

She has served in healthcare executive roles for several global companies, most recently UnitedHealthcare. Rebecca is happiest when outdoors, practicing yoga, finding great Mexican food, being a mom, and using her chaotic Aries energy for good. She was born in Bloomington, IN, grew up in Houston, TX, and has lived in Nashville, TN, since 2005.

Author photo © Chris Loomis

SELECTED TITLES FROM SHE WRITES PRESS

She Writes Press is an independent publishing company founded to serve women writers everywhere. Visit us at www.shewritespress.com.

Falling Together: How to Find Balance, Joy, and Meaningful Change When Your Life Seems to be Falling Apart by Donna Cardillo. $16.95, 978-1-63152-077-8. A funny, big-hearted self-help memoir that tackles divorce, caregiving, burnout, major illness, fears, and low self-esteem—and explores the renewal that comes when we are able to meet these challenges with courage.

Green Nails and Other Acts of Rebellion: Life After Loss by Elaine Soloway. $16.95, 978-1-63152-919-1. An honest, often humorous account of the joys and pains of caregiving for a loved one with a debilitating illness.

Hug Everyone You Know: A Year of Community, Courage, and Cancer by Antoinette Truglio Martin. $16.95, 978-1-63152-262-8. Cancer is scary enough for the brave, but for a wimp like Antoinette Martin, it was downright terrifying. With the help of her community, however, Martin slowly found the courage within herself to face cancer—and to do so with perseverance and humor.

Beautiful Affliction: A Memoir by Lene Fogelberg. $16.95, 978-1-63152-985-6. The true story of a young woman's struggle to raise a family while her body slowly deteriorates as the result of an undetected fatal heart disease.

Body 2.0: Finding My Edge Through Loss and Mastectomy by Krista Hammerbacher Haapala. An authentic, inspiring guide to reframing adversity that provides a new perspective on preventative mastectomy, told through the lens of the author's personal experience.

The First Signs of April: A Memoir by Mary-Elizabeth Briscoe. $16.95, 978-1631522987. Briscoe explores the destructive patterns of unresolved grief and the importance of connection for true healing to occur in this inspirational memoir, which weaves through time to explore grief reactions to two very different losses: suicide and cancer.